D1314016

I couldn't picture most of what we were about to see.

MARLENE TRESTMAN, ELI'S MOM

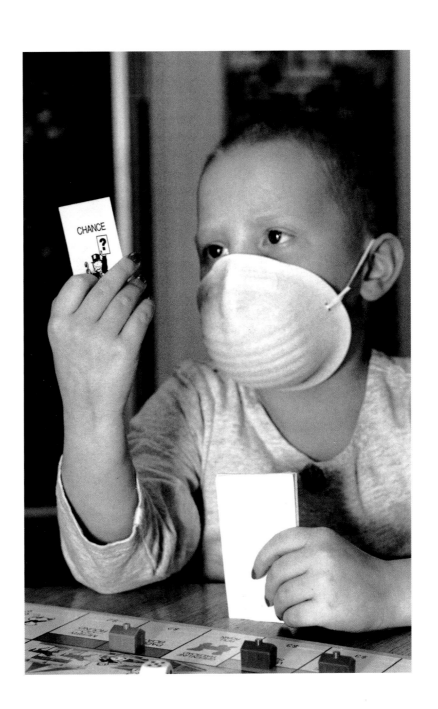

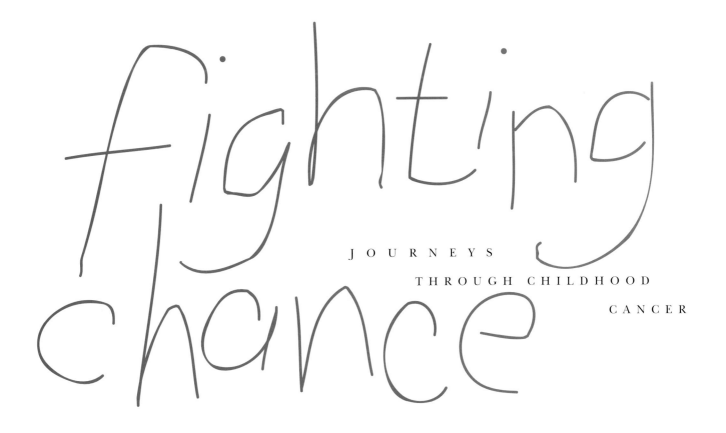

fighting chance

JOURNEYS

THROUGH CHILDHOOD

CANCER

photographs and story by

Harry Connolly

contributions by

Tom Clancy

Curt I. Civin, MD

Professor, Oncology and Pediatrics
Director, Pediatric Oncology
The Johns Hopkins University
School of Medicine

WOODHOLME
HOUSE
PUBLISHERS

Baltimore, Maryland

Printed and bound in Hong Kong.

1 2 3 4 5   06 05 04 03 02 01 00 99 98

Library of Congress Cataloging-in-Publication Data
Connolly, Harry.
    Fighting chance : journeys through childhood cancer /
photographs by Harry Connolly ;
contributions by Tom Clancy, Curt I. Civin.
    p.   cm.
ISBN 0-9656342-5-6
    1. Tumors in children—Patients—Maryland—
Baltimore—Biography. 2. Tumors in children—
Patients—Maryland—Baltimore—Pictorial works.
I. Clancy, Tom, 1947- . II. Civin, Curt I. III. Title.
RC281.C4C665 1997
362.1´9892994—dc21   97-14834
                 CIP

Woodholme House Publishers
1829 Reisterstown Road
Suite 130
Baltimore, Maryland 21208
Fax: (410) 653-7904
Orders: 1-800-488-0051

Book design: Greaney Design, Baltimore
Jacket design: Gerry Greaney
Inside flap photograph: Keith Patrick

This book is lovingly dedicated to

Eli, Heather, and Keith, my young heroes,

and to the memory of

Harry and Marion Connolly, my first heroes.

The Pediatric Oncology Department of Johns Hopkins Hospital is dedicated to saving the lives of children. A place for brilliant research and compassionate care, it is also a place of laughter and tears, wins and losses, hopes and prayers. Here, superb caregivers do the toughest of jobs with skill, courage, and amazing grace.

My thanks to everyone at Hopkins, especially Drs. Curt Civin, Michael Kastan, Maria Pelidis, and Stanton Goldman, and the 8 East staff. To the Ped. Onc. clinic, I owe a special debt.

Thanks also to: Tom Clancy, Drs. Roger Lewin and Arnold Sigler, Anne Tyler, Tom Wilson, Gary Kaich, Manuela Soares, Patricia Bittrick, Michael Feinstein, Bob Tucker, and Armand Himes for their support; Dr. Gordon Livingston, Michael Olesker, and Sharon and Lizzie Fairbrother for their inspiring stories; Thatcher Hogan of Kodak Professional and Sharon Lebowitz of Nikon USA (their films and cameras are wonderful; their support was immediate, generous, greatly appreciated); Chuck Verrill, Gregg Wilhelm, and Gerry Greaney—agent, editor, designer, friends.

The family I love: Renée, my boy, Wil, and Joey, my sisters Rosemary, Eileen, Anne, Kathleen, Caroline, and Marion, the out-laws, and all the families I met in this journey. Every child *is* special.

I am most indebted to three families: Marlene Trestman, Henry, Helene, and Eli Kahn; Phyllis Vines, Dee, Angel, and Heather Brogdon; and Bob, Dawn, Scott, and Keith Patrick. When times were tough, they said "Yes." And that made all the difference.

My "doctor's words" lack the power to capture the stories of these terrific children. Harry Connolly's beautiful pictures open up their world. Their stories have been hidden for too long. Theirs is a world of joy, like any child's, but they have been forgotten people—young kids struggling quietly to save their lives from an unfair enemy. Families have put aside careers, sold homes, sacrificed and suffered a thousand losses. For too many, all this has failed to stop their children's cancers.

Parents are sent to us unknowing. Time matters. They have to trust us. Tense, they answer our medical history questions, allow us to examine their child's small body, then freeze as we confirm their pediatrician's suspicion. We think, and later we know, that their child has cancer. Though they have only just met us, though they don't fully understand the disease, they must essentially hand their child over to us for tests and treatments they fear—blood tests, X-rays, bone marrow analyses, spinal taps, surgery, radiation therapy, chemotherapy. Their trust comes from desperate courage.

We must merit that trust. Parents want their child back...cured.

Parents often wonder what they did wrong. How did this happen? Parents must not blame themselves.

Doctors don't know exactly what causes cancer, but we have a concept. As children grow and develop, cells in their body tissues must generate many additional cells. To do this, cells divide and reproduce themselves at an incredible rate. Sometimes, these cells make a mistake in duplicating the DNA blueprint, like misspelling a word. Generally, the mistake does not matter or if the mistake is serious the cell dies. But sometimes a cell containing a big mistake continues to divide and reproduce, then another mistake occurs in one of the daughter cells. A few crucial mistakes and the cell becomes cancerous, divides, and reproduces cancerous daughter cells just like itself that cannot develop.

Leukemia and lymphoma are relatively common forms of childhood cancer. These cancers start in an early cell of the immune system. Most commonly, this cell should have developed into a B cell, a cell that makes an antibody. Instead, the leukemia cells just divide, and they crowd out normal developing blood and immune cells, as can be seen in diagnostic bone marrow samples through a microscope.

The three children in *Fighting Chance* are representative of these forms of cancer. Eli's and Heather's leukemias arose in a developing bone marrow B lymphoid cell, and spread throughout the body. Cells in bone marrow quickly go into the blood. Keith's type of cancer, a T cell lymphoma, started similarly in a developing T lymphoid cell in the thymus gland near his heart. Mature T cells provide immunity against viruses. Fortunately, when Keith was diagnosed the cancer had not spread beyond his chest.

At one time, the diagnosis of cancer in a child meant a rapid death for more than seventy percent of patients. Advances in combined modality treatment—surgery, radiation therapy, chemotherapy in precise combination—have reversed the odds. Today, nearly seventy percent of children with cancer can be cured. This has required an enormous investment, but this investment will continue forever to richly pay off. Every day, children are saved from cancers which, when I was a medical student, were uniformly fatal.

Still, thirty percent of those children entrusted to me will die. This intolerable thought motivates my research toward understanding how cancers grow. The urgent challenge is to conceive more effective and less toxic ways to diagnose, cure, and ultimately prevent cancer.

There is nothing more beautiful than seeing research lead to cures.

Today, nearly one person in every thousand in America is a survivor of childhood cancer. The molecular tools and the growing understanding that biomedical science has put at our command is incredibly powerful. The time is here to give these children an even better fighting chance of survival.

Curt I. Civin, MD

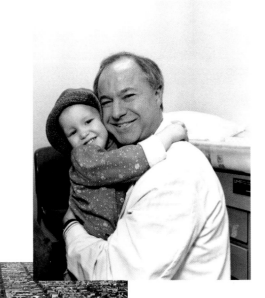

What do you do at Hopkins?

I treat children with cancer.

Oh, that must be so hard.

Why? I help to save kids' lives every day.

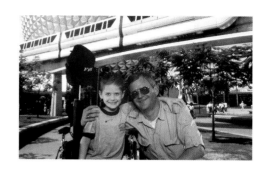

It started for me by accident. I met a little boy named Kyle, and it got very personal very fast. Six-and-a-half years old when I got to know him, eight years and twenty-six days when he died, Kyle was my little buddy—not a distant abstraction at all, a real kid, my son's age, bright and funny and perceptive...and fatally ill from the first moment I learned his name.

Personal? Pushing a dying little boy around Disney World in a wheelchair for the first/last time is just as personal as hell. You cannot be a man and not be affected by such a thing, whether he's your kid or not. Aren't we all parents to all kids? Isn't that part of the contract of adulthood? We're the ones who hug the kids when things aren't going right, and the hug makes it right again, doesn't it? Well, imagine that your hug doesn't help at all, that you make a special little friend who says to you over the phone, "Tom, when I grow up, if I live..." and then dies a week later.

Yeah, try imagining that and then you wonder about the people who do this sort of thing for a living—the medical warriors.

All wars are bad. Some are worse than others. This book is about the worst and nastiest of all. You can't see the enemy except, maybe, through a microscope. Strength of arms is useless against it because the enemy doesn't stand and fight in the open as men do. This enemy chooses its victims at random and this book is about an enemy that chooses kids as its special targets. It's about the kids who are drafted into the war against their innocent will. It's about the families and friends of the kids. It's about the warriors—physcians, scientists, nurses, medical technicians—who fight a nearly invisible foe.

The enemy is pediatric cancer, and everyone in these photos is fighting it in one way or another. The children fight back as victims who want to live normal lives in the face of this most sinister and cruelest of maladies. Throughout the war they will do their best to just be kids—just to play and watch cartoons and embrace the world as it is supposed to be for kids, a place of wonder and delight, learning and growing, love and friendship. They hold onto that reality with small but powerful hands, perhaps because as children they don't really recognize the dangers to which they ought not be exposed in the first place.

Meanwhile, all around them the best minds and tools the medical profession has evolved are marshalled like an army to fight the war within the bodies of the victims...and the children hang on to their childhood with a hard grip.

The parents hold their hands—but not too tightly lest they hurt their children more—and are there to be strong for them. They cry out of sight of their kids at the injustice of the entire nightmare, at the pain which should not be, of the childhood being stolen before their eyes, at the danger they are unable to hold back along with the other dangers from which parents are supposed to protect their children.

"It's like my hands are tied," the father of a cancer victim once told me, "and somebody is laughing at me."

The warriors come last, but in the war they come first because only they can fight this particular enemy. We've all seen the clichés of war in movies and books, but the truth of the matter is that in the worst places we find the best of us to stand and fight. The rest of us depend on them to do so.

Heroic? Consider a job where the main hazard is watching children die. The kids and their families don't volunteer. The medics do, and they go to work every day just as the rest of us go to our various jobs, but it is they who must stand and fight multiple battles in this war. The things the parents and friends cannot do, the medics must. It's not just a job for them. Medicine offers many fields, all of them necessary, all of them helpful to people in need, but none so demanding as this one.

The patients have names and faces and little laughs and larger dreams all of which must be protected. But they can't all be saved, and the medics come into the job every day knowing that today might be the last for a patient whom science and luck have failed. The medics come even so. They're even cheerful. They plan to win every battle they fight, and eventually the big one.

"I'm going to get this dragon," I heard one doctor say when recruiting talented new docs. "Come follow me and be there for the kill."

He meant it. His eyes are on the prize, and he expects to win the final victory. But along the way the road to a victory not yet won is strewn with the graves of babies as the docs close in on the dragon in retreat, but not yet quite dead.

It's getting better. Childhood cancer is no longer the death sentence it was only a few years ago. The docs are getting smarter. The heroics of previous generations of kids and families and medics have paid off. If the war is nasty, at least it is no longer one-sided, and the dragon is in retreat, and so this book is one of hope.

Papa Hemingway said that courage is grace under pressure. Well, there's a lot of that in this book.

In these photos you will see the battle as it is fought, daily, mainly out of sight of most of us, but being fought even so. And it is fought for all of us, because I believe saving the life of a single child is the salvation of the entire world.

Tom Clancy

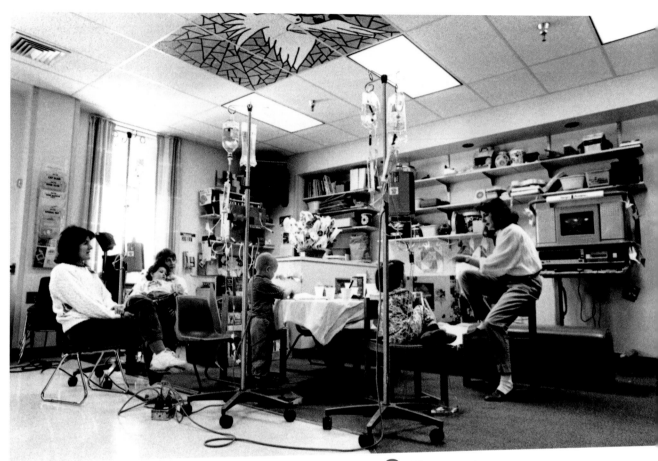

8 East

Why spend three years documenting the lives of children battling cancer? You are holding my answer in your hands. Children are a gift—to ourselves, to the future. A part of our legacy, our hopes, and our dreams go with them. At times, we ask too much of them. What we want for them is simple: a healthy and happy childhood; time to grow and learn, to play and prosper. Time to be a kid.

But cancer changes everything.

As the eye of the cancer storm rages within a child, its effects are far reaching. For the family, the world is turned upside down. Quickly, they must learn about this disease and make life or death decisions. There will be more questions than answers, but with luck, that will change. They must see what kind of childhood is still possible. Win or lose, nothing will ever be the same.

As family and friends rally in support, others will disappear, unwilling or unable to help. The greatest help may be found in a hospital. There, using the best science at their disposal, doctors and their staffs initiate treatments and procedures. Their goal is simple, ruthless: Kill the cancer, save the child.

There are few people whose lives have not been touched by cancer. I am no exception. My father was a surgeon who loved his medicine, his hospital, his patients. But he couldn't help the one he loved the most. My mother died of cancer when she was only fifty-one. I was eighteen, a part of her legacy. Her death changed everything.

The inspiration for this book came many years later. In a magazine, a boy's snapshot illustrated a father's story of his son's brave, but futile, fight against cancer. Taken by his mother, enlarged to fill the page, the snapshot's flaws are revealed. All wrong, yet so right. Out of focus, mother and son moved as the shutter clicked. You see the blue eyes, the wild blonde hair, the boyish expression—but you feel his spirit. One moment in a brief life. It filled me with sadness and wonder. Feeling the pull of this picture, I ripped it out of the magazine.

Months later, it led me to Dr. Curt Civin and the Pediatric Oncology Department of Johns Hopkins Hospital in Baltimore, Maryland. There, knowing little about the world of childhood cancer, I started this story. Hopkins' pediatric oncology unit is in The Children's Center, on the eighth floor, east wing. Walking the 8 East hall for the first time, I knew I was heading into uncharted territory. Asking strangers to let me follow their children. In and out of the hospital. Asking doctors and staff to let me into their world. Asking everyone to trust me. Come what may. Good times or bad; remission, relapse, or cure. Life or death. None of us could say where this journey would lead.

When I discovered that Lucas, the boy in the magazine, had been a Hopkins patient, I knew I was in the right place. His photograph guided me to 8 East, to the floor where a boy and his family had fought and lost their battle. One circle completed.

Our journey is about to begin.

Harry Connolly

Having a child develop a malignancy is like being struck by lightning. It's that rare.

DR. MICHAEL KASTAN

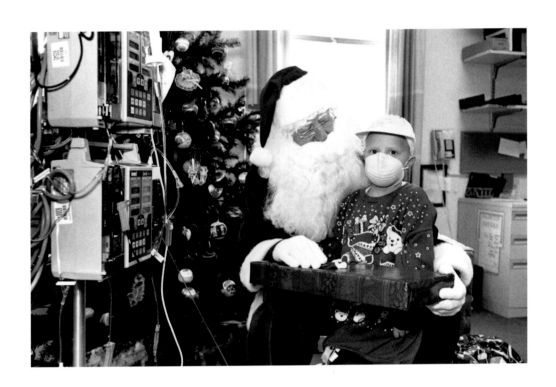

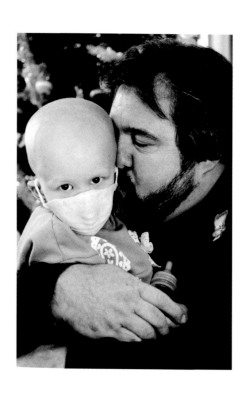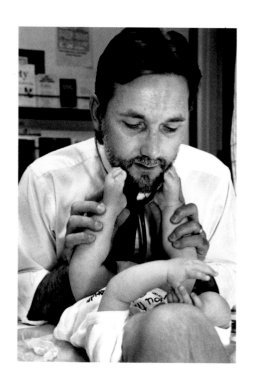

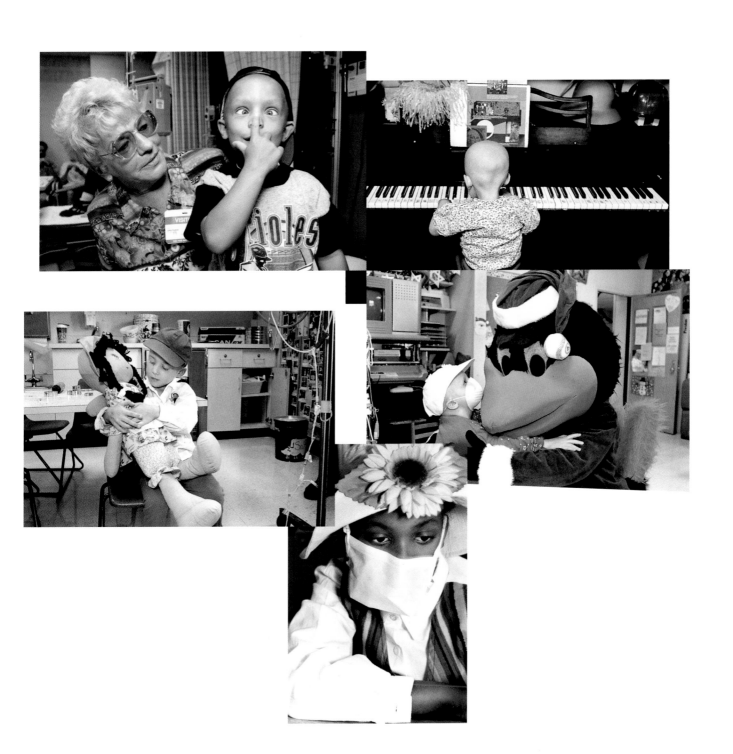

Keith

The halls are decorated and a Christmas party sprinkles a little cheer throughout 8 East. In the playroom sit kids who must stay in the hospital, those who can't go home for the holidays. There is pizza and punch, cookies and sodas. The doctors wear holiday ties. The nursing staff sports holiday sweatshirts and jewelry. Santa hats are passed around the room. After visits by the Baltimore Oriole mascot and Barney the Dinosaur, Santa Claus arrives with his sack full of presents.

Despite everyone's best efforts, joy is in short supply. No one wants to be here. It seems hardest on parents, who want their children to be healthy, happy, and at home. They also want to be happy, but that may be impossible. Still, the adults try their best and the children respond. They appreciate the presents, the hugs, the love and attention.

The boy I am looking for is not at the party. I find Keith in his room, asleep by the window. He is sixteen, just back from port implant surgery where a line for chemotherapy was inserted in his chest. Wrapped in white sheets and a hospital gown, he looks like a disheveled angel. Quickly, quietly, I photograph this boy, this stranger. Not knowing his disease, his prognosis, or whether he will let me follow him, I do know that this moment cannot be repeated.

I meet his parents and learn that just two days ago, by phone, Dawn and Bob Patrick learned that their youngest son might have cancer. While their doctor can't be certain of his diagnosis, he is sure that Keith needs further tests. Yesterday, they left their Maryland farm to travel eighty-five miles to a city they had visited only once, to a hospital they had never before seen.

In the noisy clinic, Keith is too upset to talk. His nurse, Teresa Sweeney, tells him, "It's okay, I'll do the talking for both of us. I'll take care of you." Teresa helps Keith and his parents through that day as they learn of Keith's T cell lymphoma.

I ask Dawn and Bob if I may follow their son. I explain to them what I plan to do. The problem is I really have no idea what I plan to do. This is "day one." I am asking a great deal of them. Tired and worried, still they are polite. "It's up to Keith."

They don't think he'll agree, but they will ask. I, too, have doubts. I worry that, at age sixteen, he is too old. Time will prove me wrong and Keith will surprise his parents.

He will let me come along for the ride.

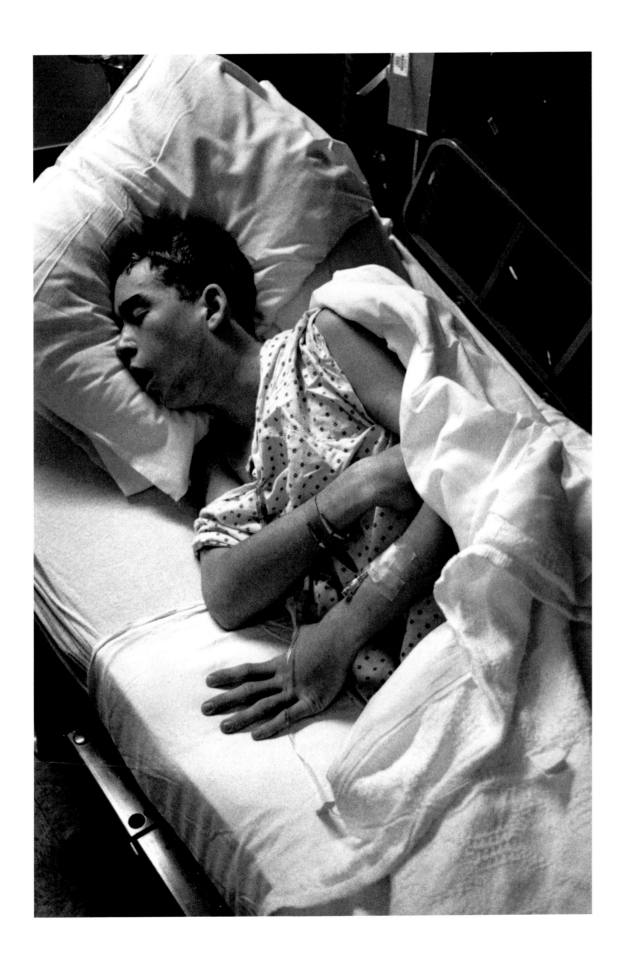

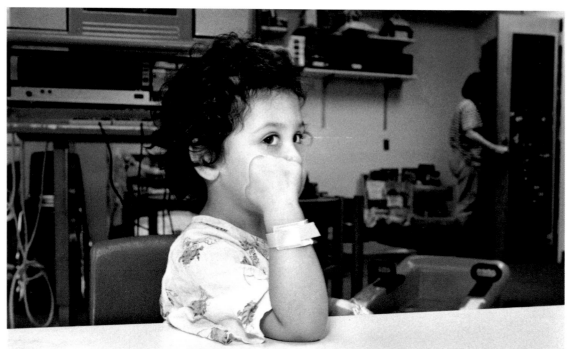

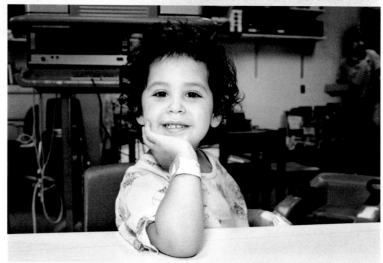

Eli

Wouldn't it be great if we could save some of these kids?

DR. ARNOLD SIGLER, RESIDENT, JOHNS HOPKINS HOSPITAL, 1960

Thirty years ago, the question was not whether a child with cancer would die, but when? Thirty years later, Dr. Arnold Sigler examines a young boy. Eli Kahn, two-and-a-half years old, has a low-grade fever and no energy. Having fallen out of bed several nights ago, he walks with a limp. His parents, Henry and Marlene, expect Dr. Sigler can treat their son. But, as Dr. Sigler examines Eli, an alarm sounds in his head. Small signs, intuition, and experience lead him to suspect a bigger problem. "At Hopkins," he says, "I was taught to be a bit of a sleuth." He takes Eli's blood, and sends mother and son home to their suburban Baltimore neighborhood. That evening, he looks at the blood smears, finds "just a few" malignant cells that confirm his suspicions, and makes two phone calls. First he phones a colleague at Johns Hopkins Hospital to arrange an immediate appointment for Eli. Then he calls Henry and Marlene to tell them that their only son has Acute Lymphocytic Leukemia (ALL), the most common of all childhood cancers.

Winter—one of the worst on record—has just begun. Tonight, one family receives news they never expected. In a moment, their world is pulled inside out. The next weeks promise a cruel introduction to the world of childhood cancer: hospital visits, overnight stays, complications. Their son will undergo procedures and begin chemotherapy. As the days run together, their emotions will ride the rollercoaster. Matters once thought important become trivial. Work will be set aside or forgotten. The Kahns will meet other families involved in similar struggles and forge friendships—comrades in arms.

Prior to morning rounds, the 8 East medical staff meets in the conference room. Covering a range of medical and emotional issues, they detail the status of each child: diagnosis and prognosis, complete blood counts, complications, yesterday's wins and losses. Their vocabulary is mysterious: ANCs, T cells, neuroblastoma, neutropenia, Methotrexate, bone marrow transplant, lumbar puncture. Occasionally, familiar words filter through: leukemia, lymphoma, remission, hospice, home, bereavement. At times, their voices indicate how a particular child is doing. Often, their faces say it all.

After the conference, rounds begin. Wheelchairs and carts holding machines, laundry, odds and ends, clutter the linoleum-tiled hallway. The nurses' station is awash in forms, papers, books, computers. Above this apparent chaos is order: a board lists each patient, their diagnosis, their age, primary and secondary nurses, and their doctors.

Along one wall are two boards holding several hundred snapshots of the children of 8 East: boys in Little League uniforms and football jerseys; girls going to parties, all dressed up; children in happier times with Mickey Mouse at Disney World, with family at the beach, sitting on Santa's lap. Some of the pictures were taken here: kids celebrating their birthday, eating pizza while connected to IV pumps, pulling down their masks to make faces at the photographer. Little is private here; little is hidden.

Along another wall is a map of the world. Above it, a cartoon character asks, "If you could get on a plane or catch a boat, where would you go?" The children here are from many countries, cities, and states, but they all have the same travel plans. To speed over the miles, to be home in a heartbeat.

Most of the small rooms are shared by two children, kept company by a parent or relative day and night. These children are rarely alone. Morning rounds run early and the children are still asleep. Their parents, in reclining chairs, try to rest. Doctors examine each child thoroughly, gently. Parents' questions and concerns are addressed with startling honesty. Telling the truth is important here.

In room 831, I meet Eli, his family, and Drs. Michael Kastan and Maria Pelidis. After rounds, I return to ask Henry and Marlene for permission to follow their son through the course of his treatment. In their place, I would say "no," but they agree.

As I start to photograph Eli, in hospital, Marlene makes a request. She wants me to photograph Eli at home. Soon. "Before he loses his hair to chemotherapy."

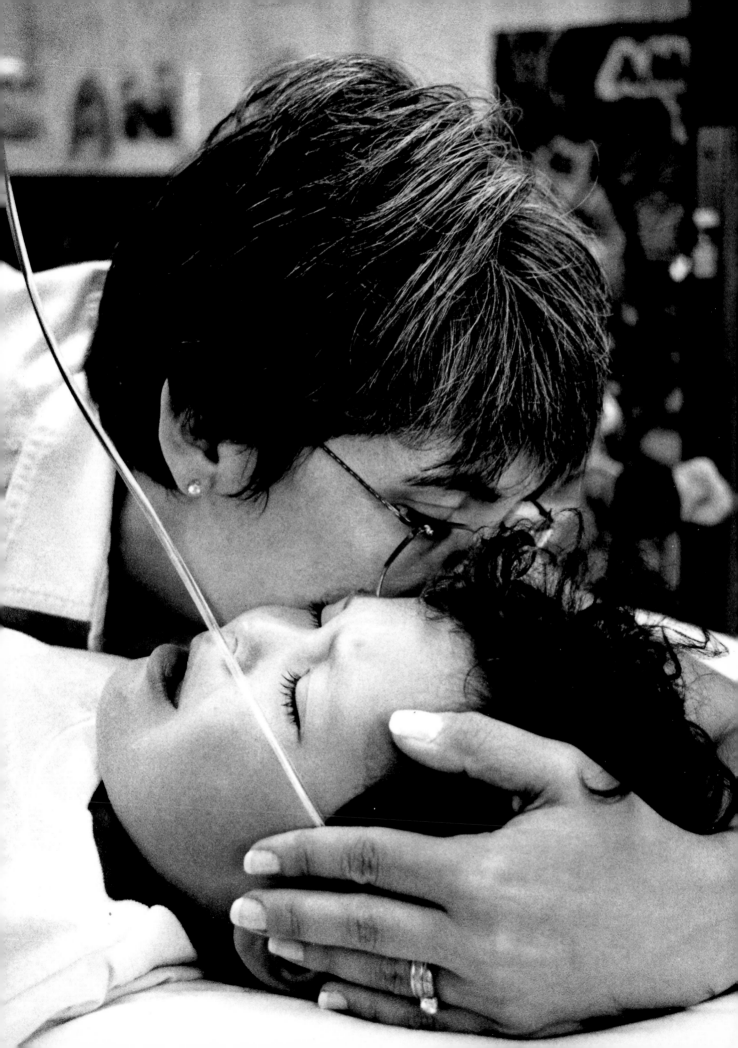

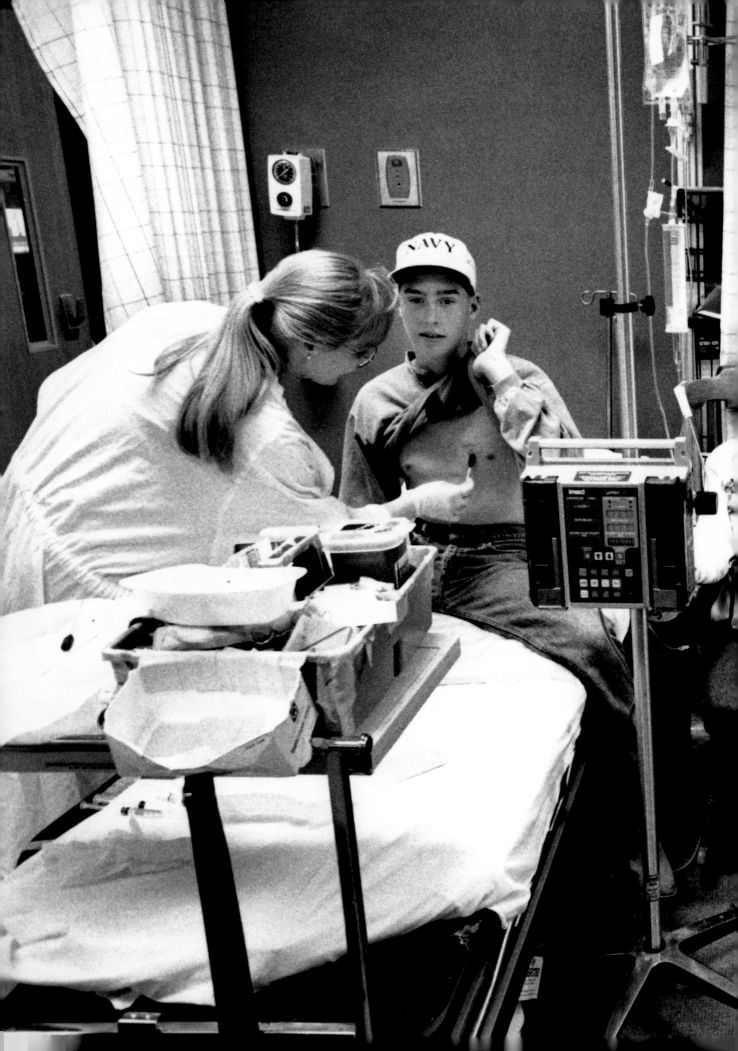

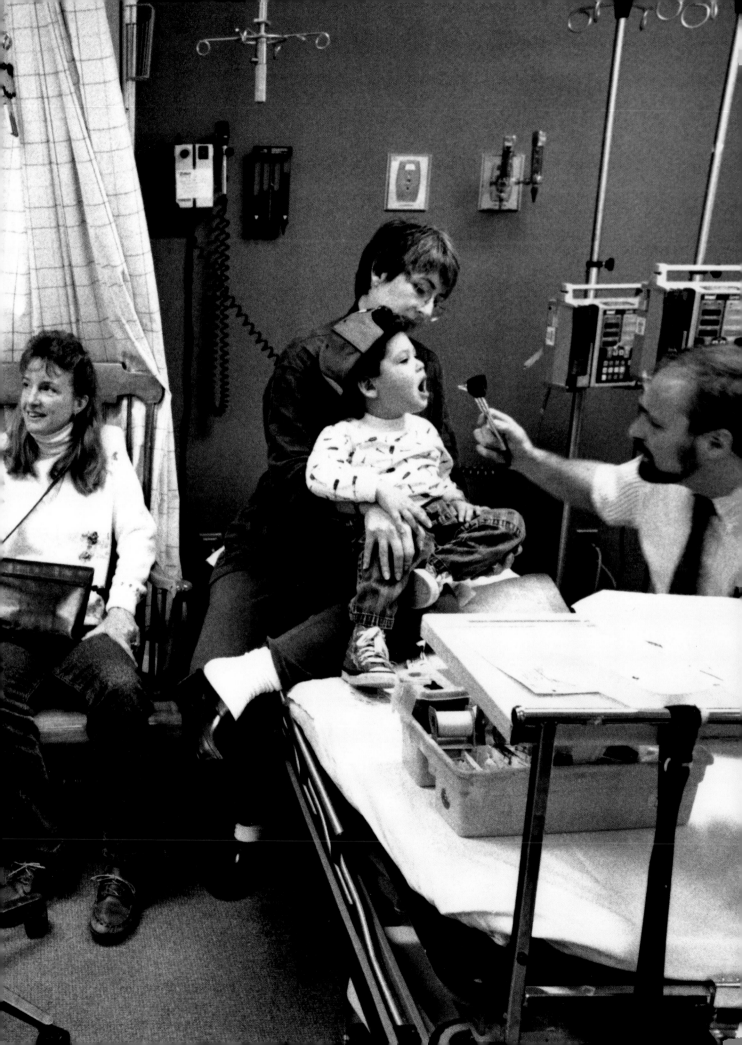

Heather

Heather Brogdon lives with her mother and two sisters in a rowhouse on a dead-end street in the city. At nine years old, Heather is the youngest child. Her father just left the family. To make ends meet, her mom, Phyllis Vines, works as much as possible.

Missing her father, Heather sits around the house crying. She won't ride her new bike. Tired, lethargic, short of breath, she loses her balance at times. She looks fragile and thin. Her mother suspects depression and something more. She thinks, "My daughter is fading away right before my eyes and I don't know what to do to save her."

Whenever Heather is ill, she goes to the nearest emergency room. This time the doctors suspect mononucleosis, but when they take her blood they seem concerned. Phyllis thinks Heather's blood looks like red Kool-Aid. When her blood is drawn a second time, Phyllis overhears two nurses whispering about cancer cells. Taken into a private room, she is told that there are cancer cells in Heather's blood, and that they must go to Johns Hopkins Hospital for further evaluation and treatment.

Trying to protect her daughter, if only for a few more hours, Phyllis keeps this news to herself.

It's after midnight when they meet Dr. Stan Goldman at Hopkins. A first year fellow, on call nearly all the time, he is tired but kind. Seeing a child for the first time, he says, "You hope for little things. You hope this is ALL (Acute Lymphocytic Leukemia), not AML (Acute Myeloid Leukemia), because her prognosis would be better."

Blood is drawn. IVs are begun. A bone marrow sample is taken. The diagnosis is made, a protocol selected, and Heather, the healthiest child in her family, is suddenly a cancer patient. Like Eli, Heather has ALL, but she has a very high number of leukemia cells. Her cancer may be harder to defeat.

Dr. Goldman tries to reassure Phyllis: "You did not cause this. This cancer could not have been prevented. There's a good chance that Heather will live."

But tonight, Phyllis finds no comfort in his words.

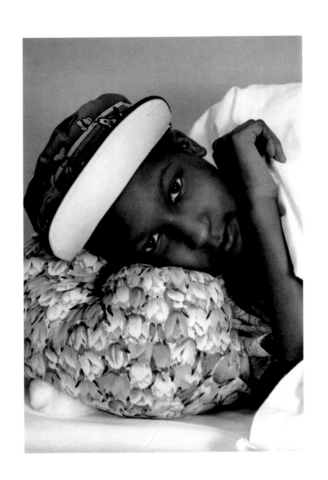

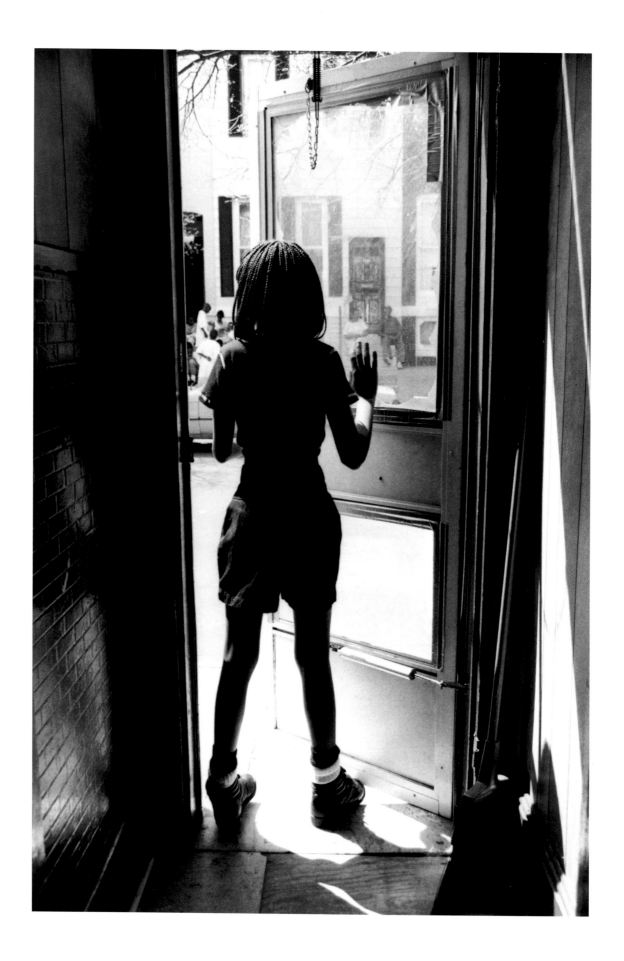

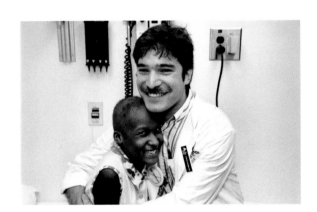

I hope I never have to appreciate how these parents

must deal with their own flesh and blood,

their own kid, having a potentially fatal disease.

It's got to be the worst feeling in the world.

It must be harder for them than for the child.

DR. STANTON GOLDMAN

All About Leukemia

BY HELENE KAHN, AGE 8

When I was only five my brother, Eli, got diagnosed with leukemia and I was really scared.
I didn't know what was going to happen.
If anyone in your family has leukemia here are some things you should know.
I'd think about all the good times like when I was in kindergarten
the whole entire class drew pictures of things Eli liked, like Barney and Baby-Bop,
and made a book out of the pictures.
We tied it with a pretty red ribbon and I took it to the hospital.
It made me feel really really good and it made Eli feel really good, too.

There was a very important car ride.
I was asking my mom questions like if either of my parents were going to get leukemia.
Another question was if Eli was going to die. I was really glad that the answers were "no."

On every other Thursday, Friday, and Saturday,
Eli would have to spend the night at the hospital and my mom stayed with Eli.
My dad and I used to bring Chinese food or pizza
and we would all go into the family room and play video games.
That made me feel really good because I was helping my own little brother
get through a horrible disease.

Every Thursday Eli had to get shots at home in his leg.
Eli thought the shot was going to hurt, then I asked Eli if he wanted me to hold his hand.
Then after the idea I had Eli got better and better at not crying.

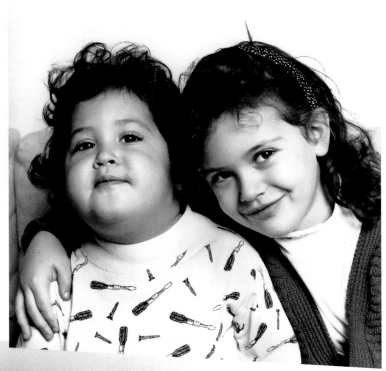

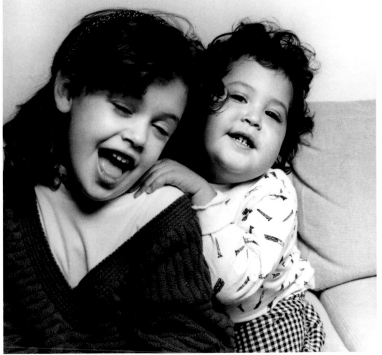

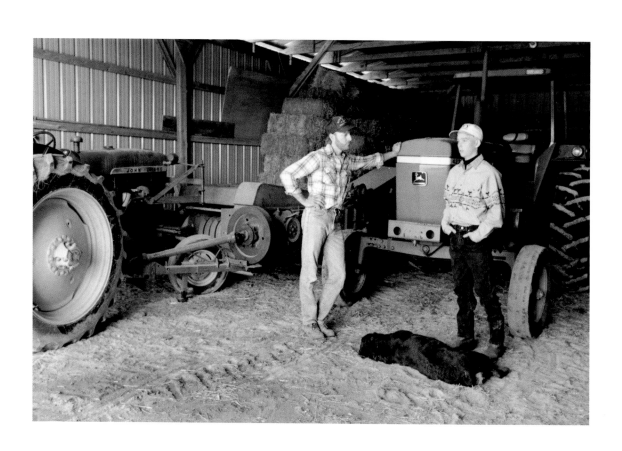

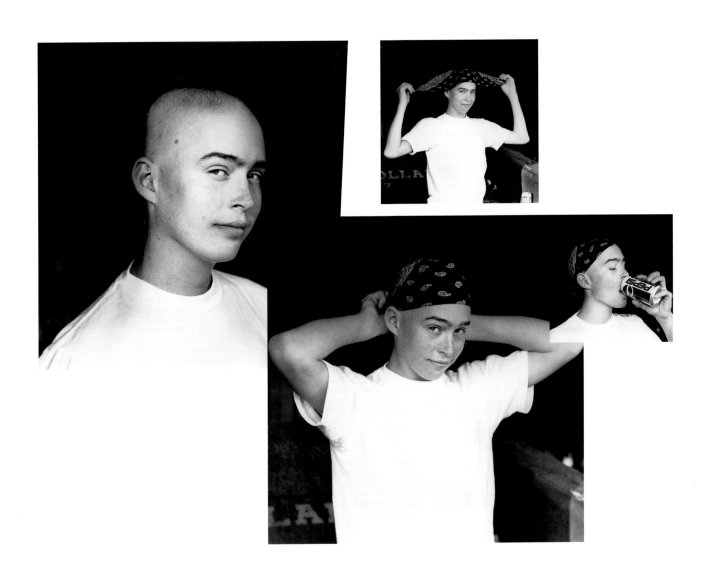

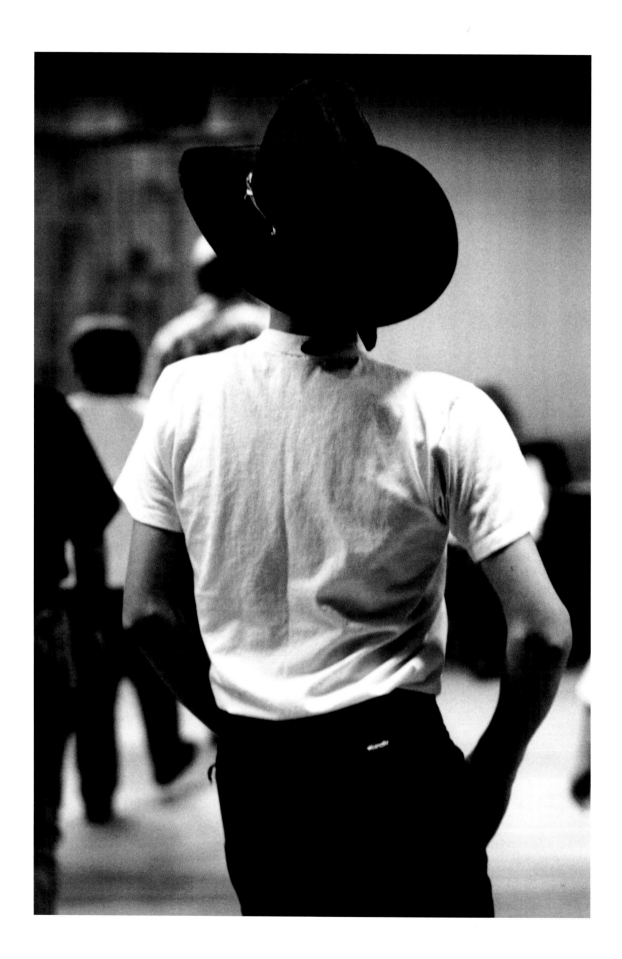

Everybody thinks they have a lot of friends, but you don't.

You only have close friends.

When you get cancer, some of your friends become acquaintances.

Different people act differently.

My best friend wants to take the pain for me.

So does my dad.

Some people are scared of me, can't look at me, talk to me.

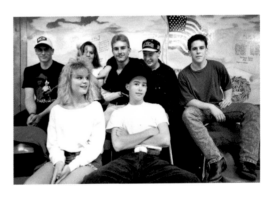

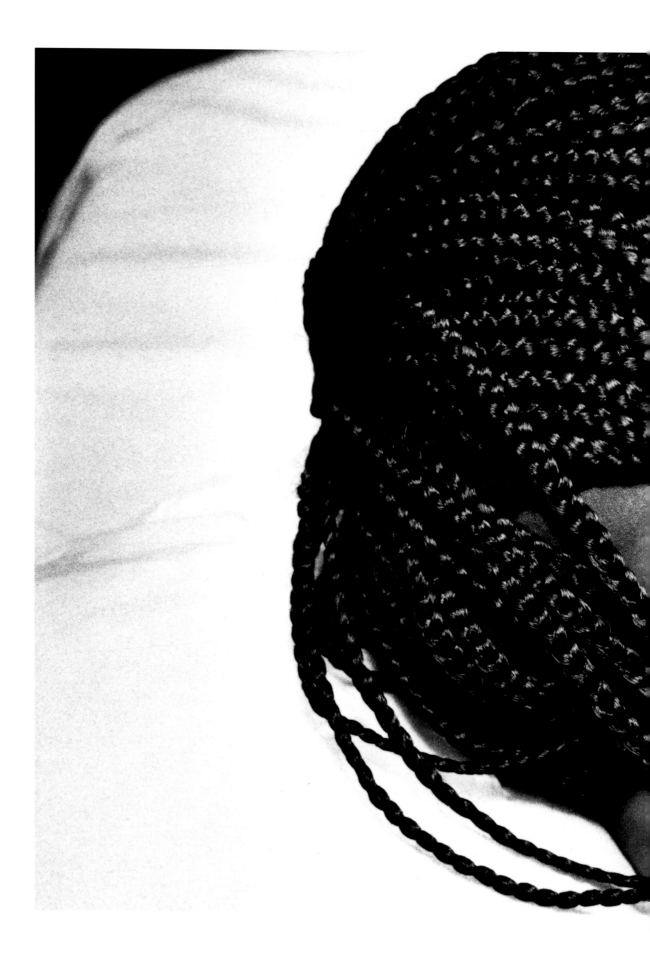

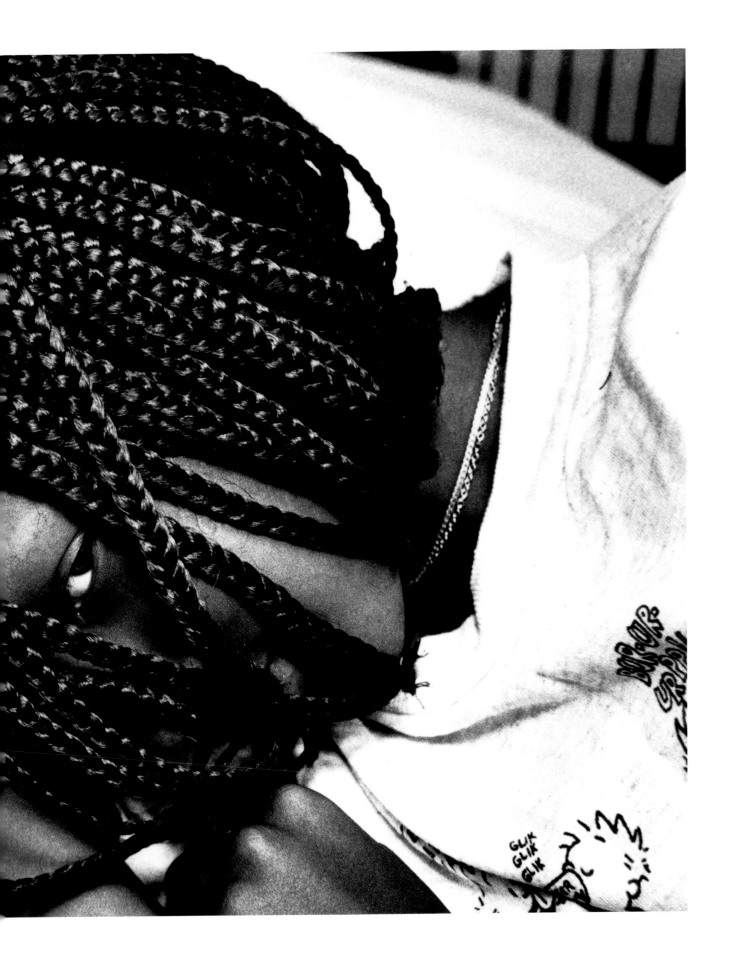

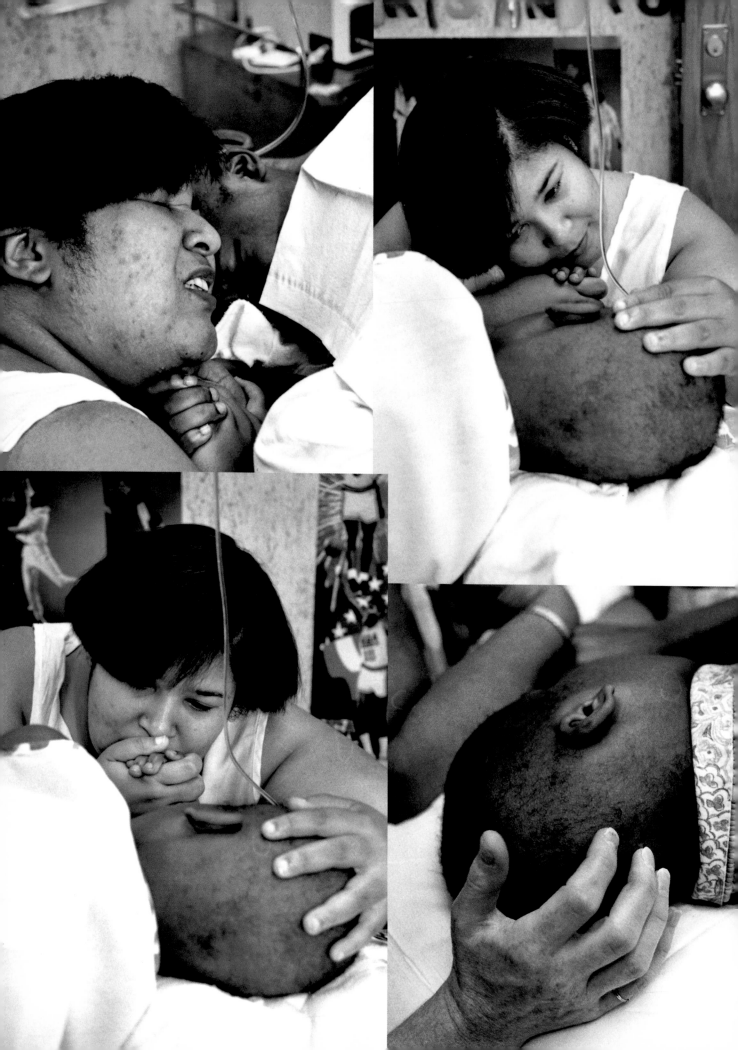

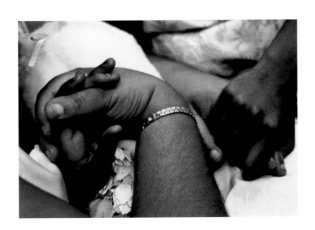

When I found out that I had leukemia,

it was very hard.

I wondered, "Why me?"

For anyone who gets leukemia,

all I am saying is stay strong and believe in yourself,

God, and your family.

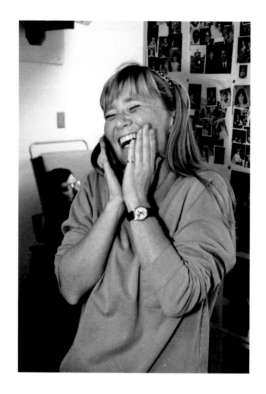

TERESA SWEENEY, RN

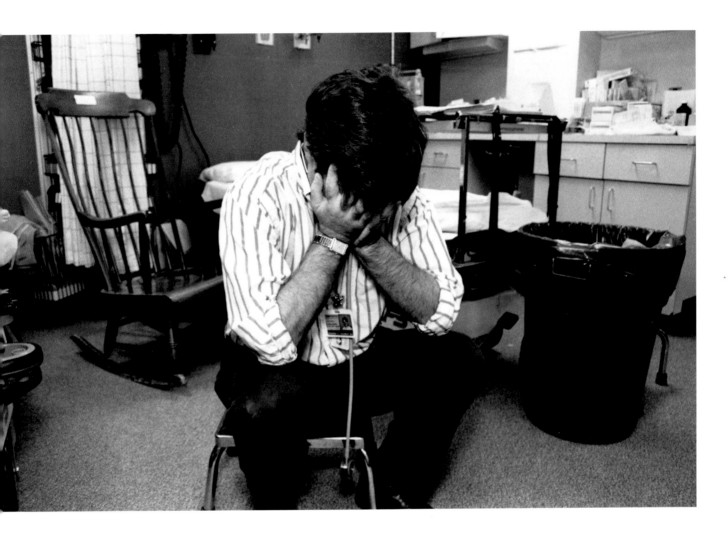

These are the most challenging kids,

the most rewarding families,

and you get the chance to make a difference

in the children's and families' lives.

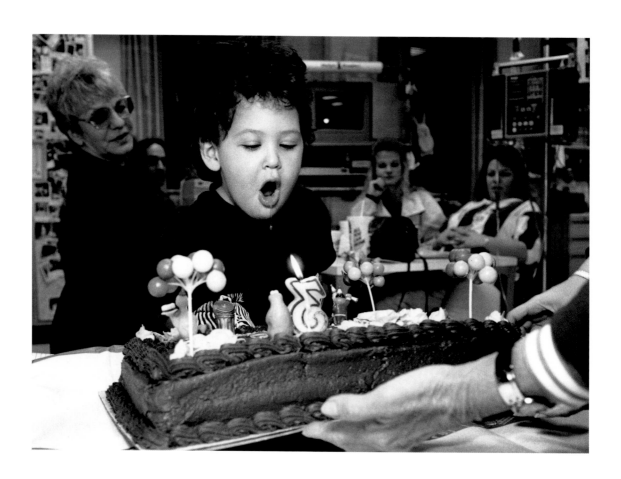

Cancer diagnoses are made through biopsies or by using two procedures that become routine throughout treatment: bone marrow analysis and spinal tap. The bone marrow test reveals the leukemia. The spinal tap shows if the cancer has gone to the spinal fluid. If so, it will be treated more aggressively. By looking at the cancer cell, doctors determine whether it is a "good" or "bad" cancer and select the best protocol or treatment plan.

Cancer cells divide rapidly. At diagnosis, a child may have a trillion cancer cells. Initial chemotherapeutic drug treatments are designed to attack these fast growing cells and reduce the number of cancer cells a thousandfold. But the cancer is still there, still deadly. More chemotherapy is required.

Eli will receive a standard risk protocol with low toxicity and high cure rates. For the first seven months he will be in the hospital for two days every two weeks. Afterwards, he'll return to the clinic for another two years of chemotherapy. Heather will undergo a high-risk treatment. Complications will lengthen the time needed to complete her protocol. Keith will receive the most aggressive protocol, enduring ten nine-week cycles of inpatient and outpatient care.

There are many side effects to chemotherapy: nausea, fever, chills, aches, hair loss, lethargy, constipation, and diarrhea. Low blood counts may lead to a higher risk of infection. Side effects vary from child to child. Early on, they will all gain weight but it will be most evident in Eli, who gains twelve pounds in a matter of weeks. All three develop mouth sores, making eating difficult—especially for Keith. "We ate tuna casseroles forever. Everyone ate it. It wasn't spicy, wasn't hard to chew. It was salty. Chemo food."

Chemotherapy's long term effects may include social and psychological difficulties, growth and reproductive problems, learning disabilities. As more children survive cancer, doctors and researchers are trying to reduce the impact these treatments have on young lives.

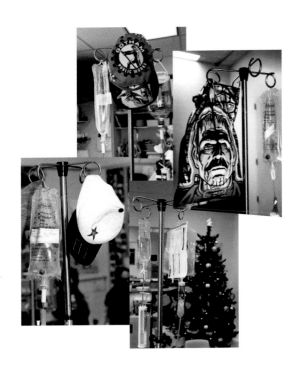

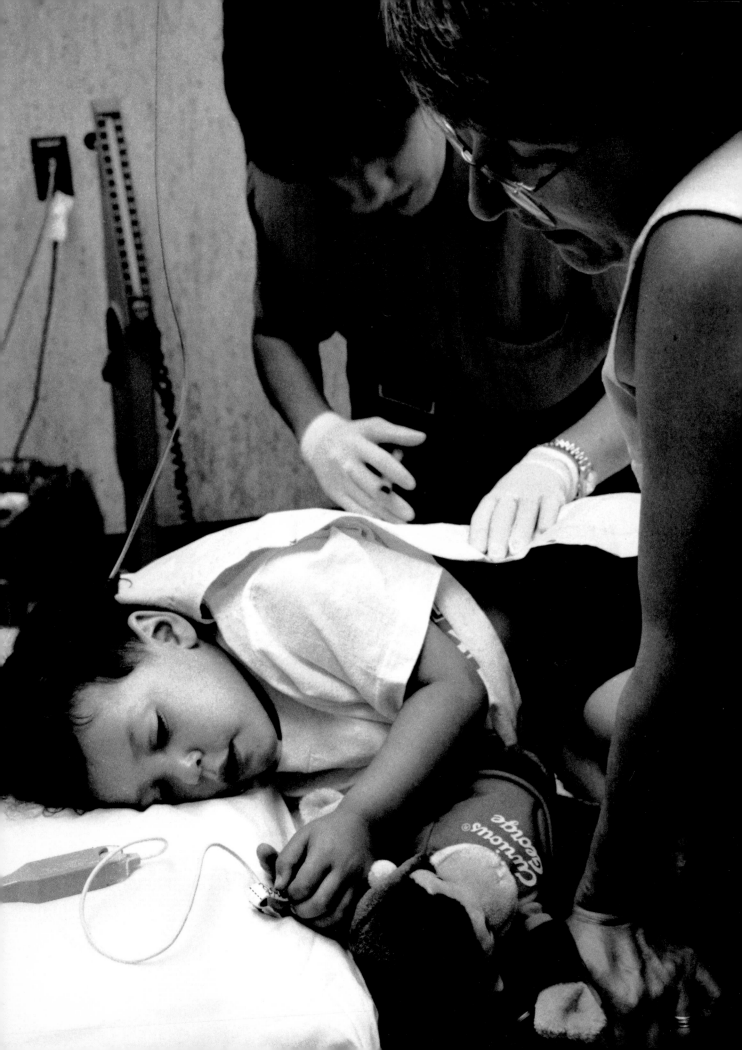

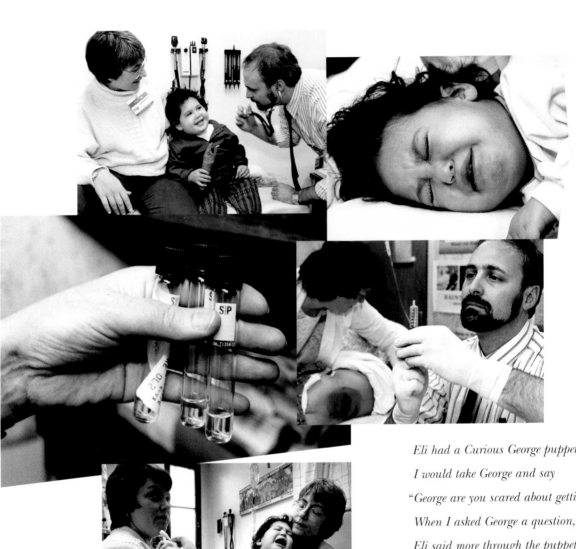

Eli had a Curious George puppet.

I would take George and say

"George are you scared about getting the shots?"

When I asked George a question,

Eli said more through the puppet

than he would on his own.

MARLENE

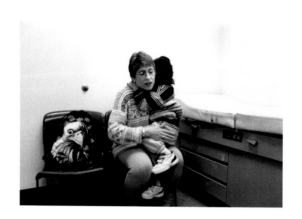

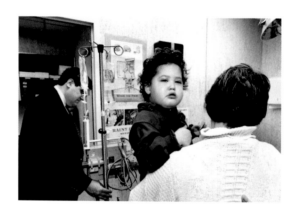

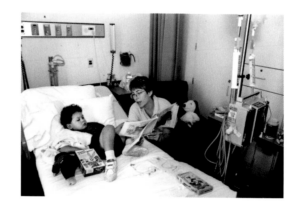

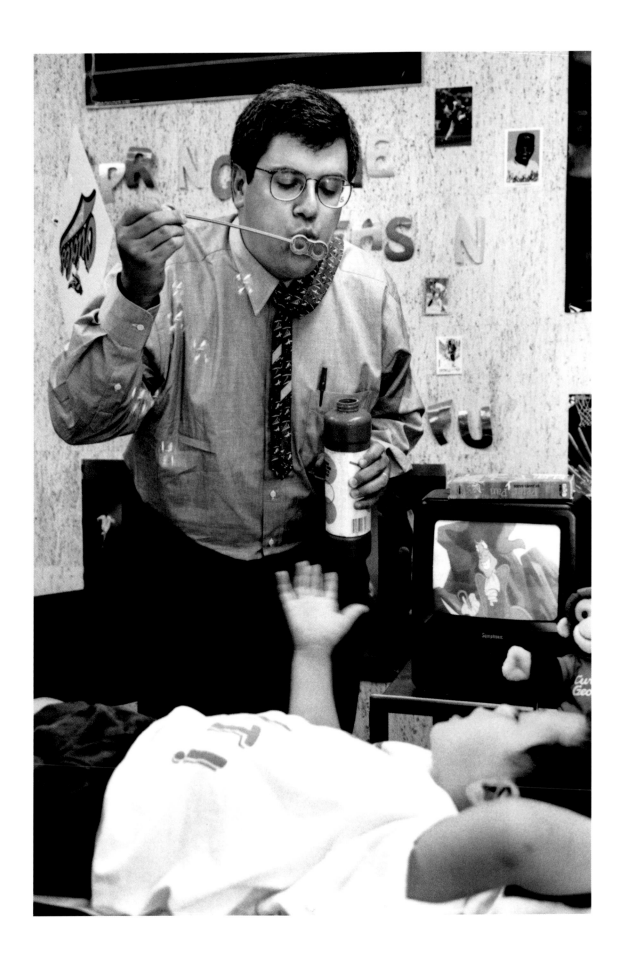

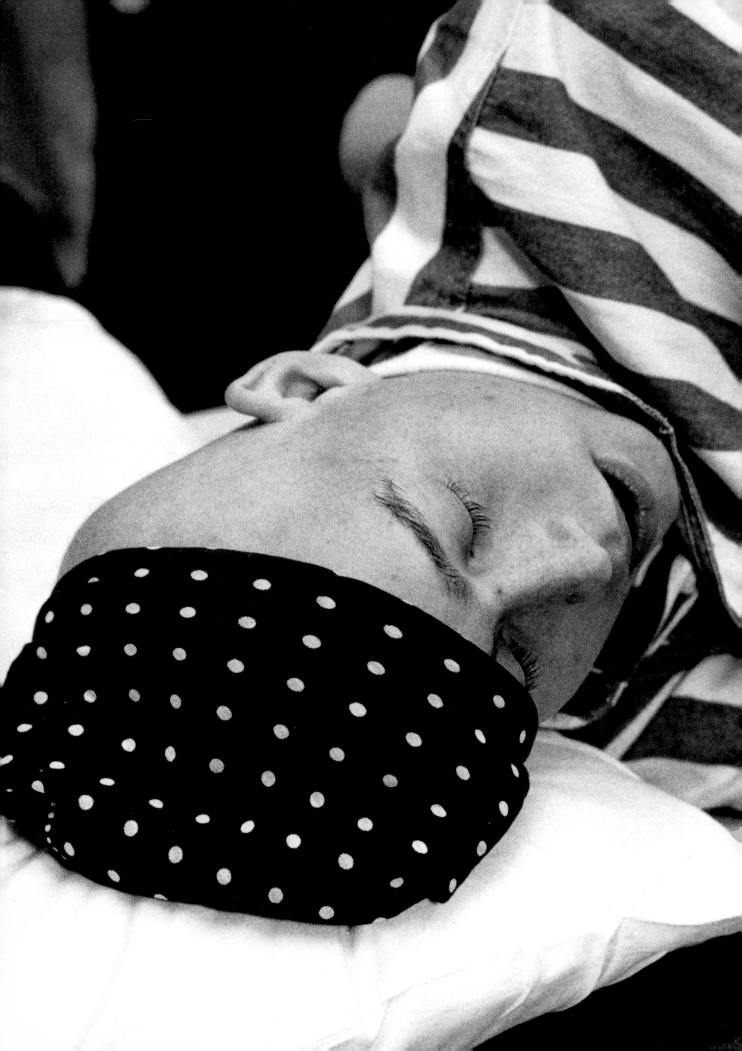

After a while, when you are talking to your tenth family whose kid has cancer,

you're more fluent in what you're going to say.

Eventually, you get to know pretty quickly what information a family can process tonight,

just enough info to help them and calm them and help the child get care.

Leave all the rest for another day.

Soon enough parents are giving shots and accessing lines.

DR. GOLDMAN

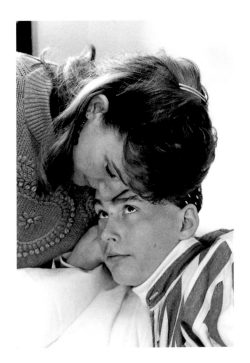

Welcome to hell.

Your life sucks from now on.

KEITH

We were numb.

They came on with a whole lot of information.

It was confusing and overwhelming.

They gave us pamphlets and books.

They told us to ask questions and eventually we would begin to understand.

We had to memorize all the drugs.

They want you to know all of the side effects.

They want you to know everything.

DAWN PATRICK

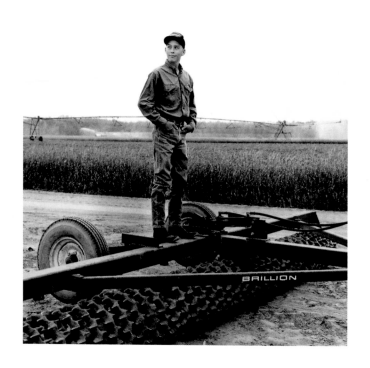

There is little talk of the future
until Keith and his dad buy a '53 Chevy truck to
restore, to paint purple, to name "Plum Hot."

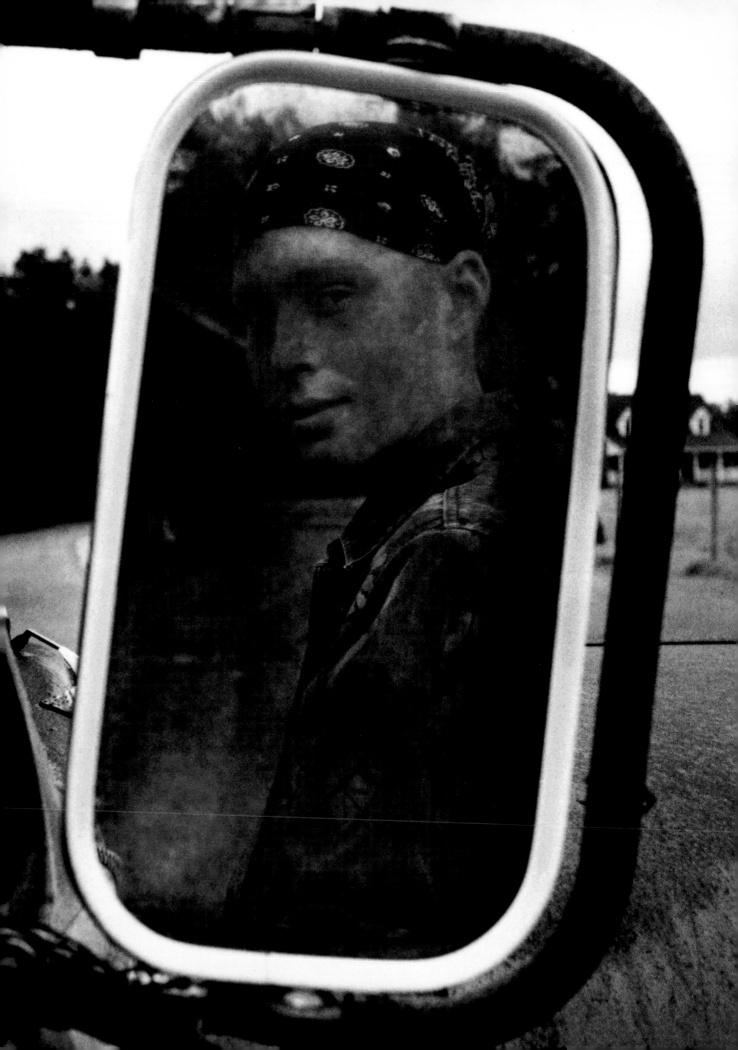

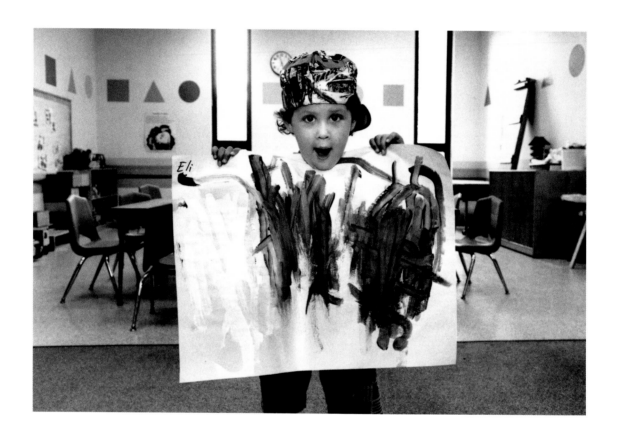

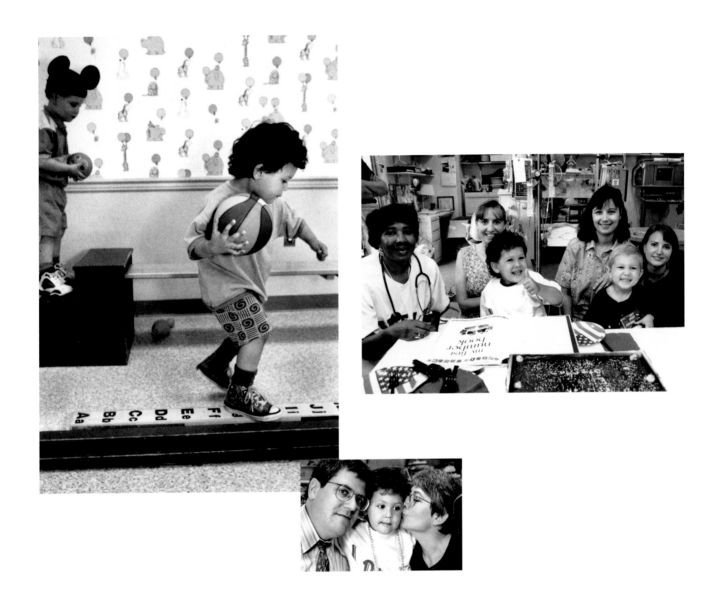

Half a year after diagnosis, Eli's inpatient treatments are complete.

However, chemotherapy continues, but it will be less toxic.

No more days in the hospital.

No more nights away from home—only visits to the hospital's clinic for treatments.

When a child reaches this milestone, 8 East throws

an "end of chemo" party with cake, ice cream, and juice for everyone.

Eli is given a baseball glove, a book, and, most importantly,

the "I Did It" t-shirt that every "end of chemo" child receives.

For the doctors, it's a chance to offer congratulations

to the Kahns. For the nurses, it's a chance to hug Eli and to say goodbye.

If all goes well, Eli will never return to 8 East.

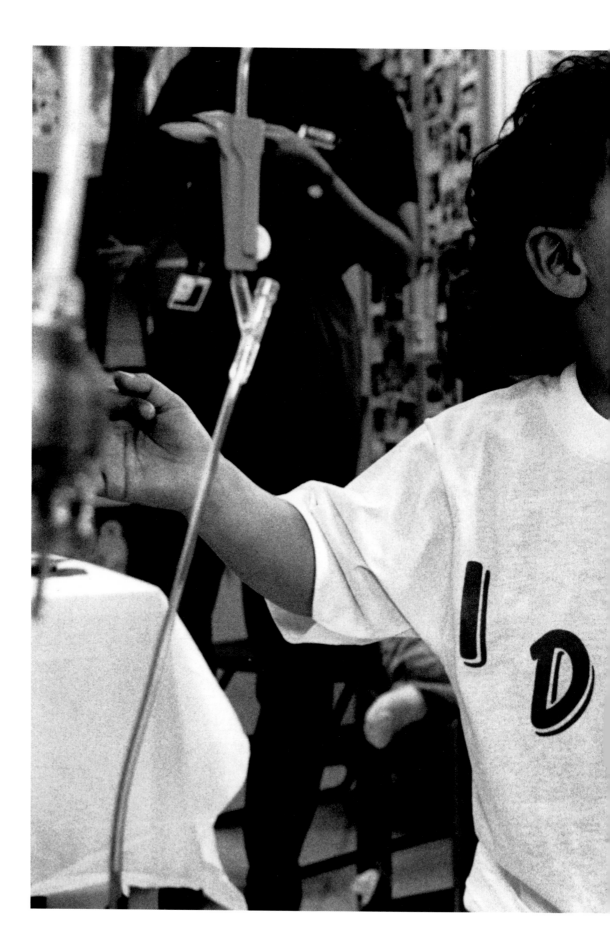

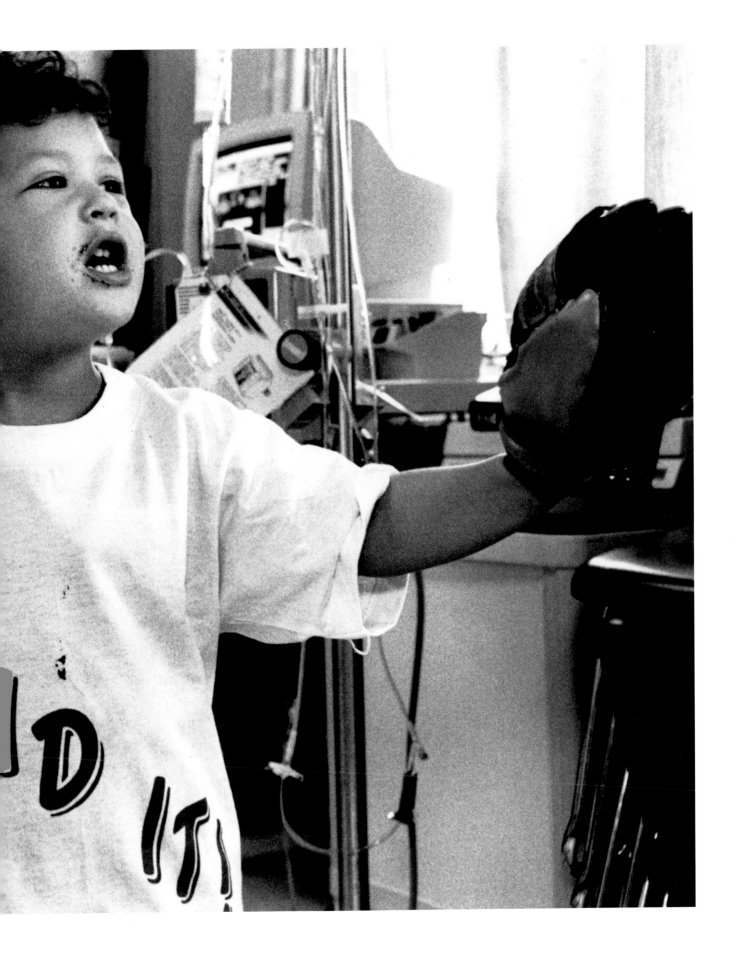

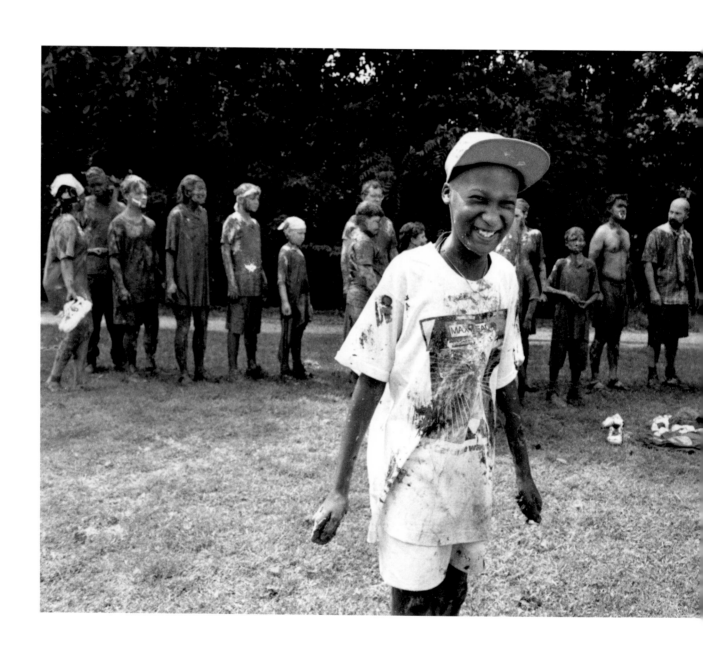

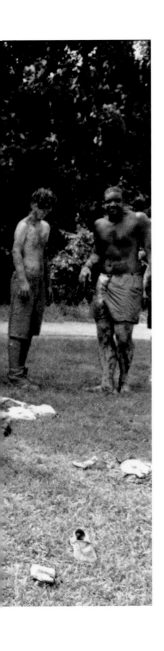
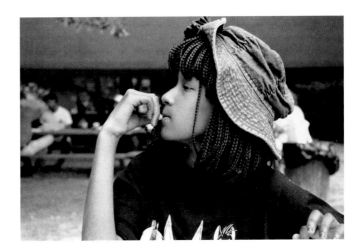

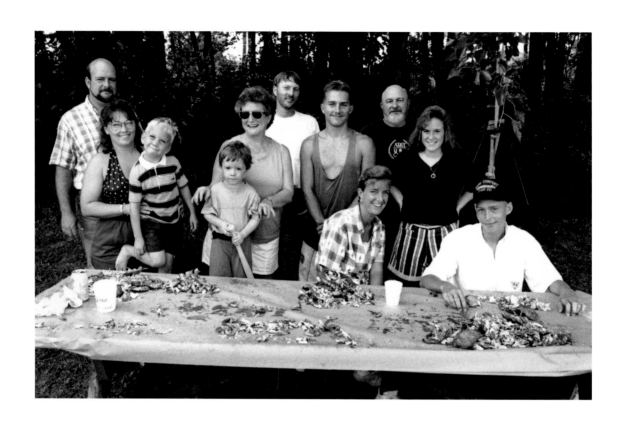

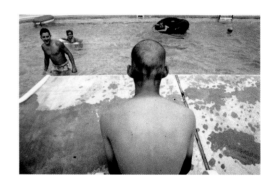

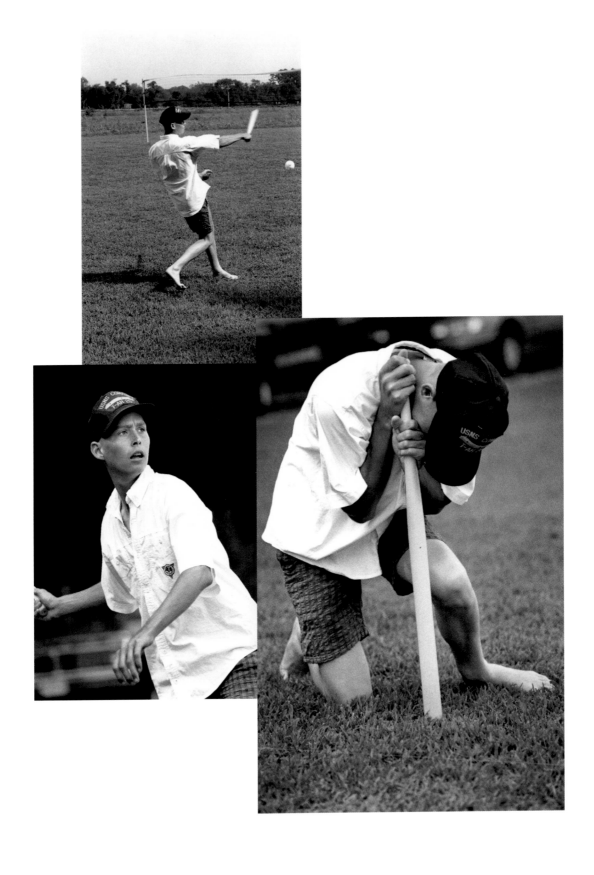

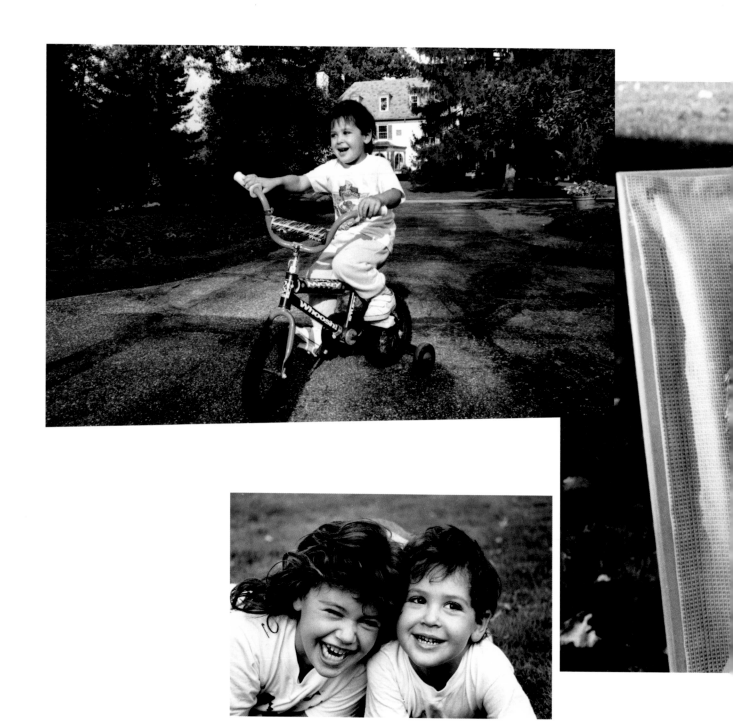

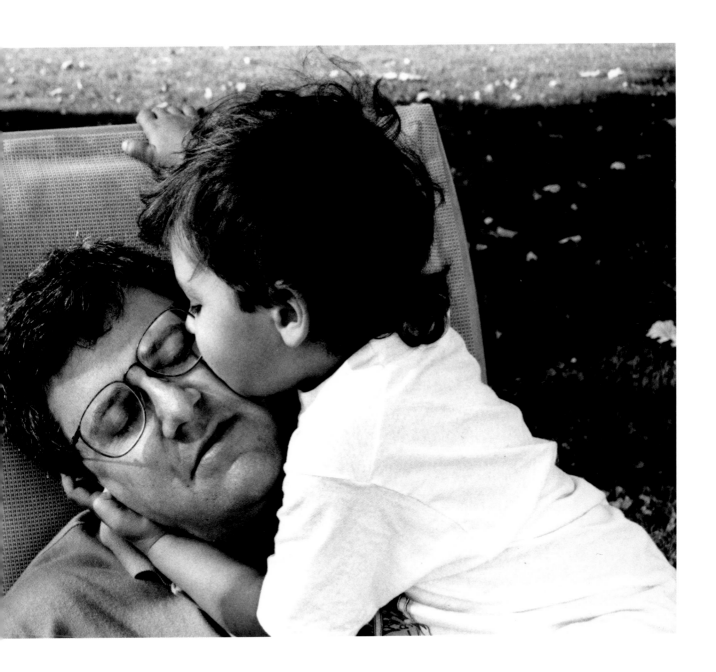

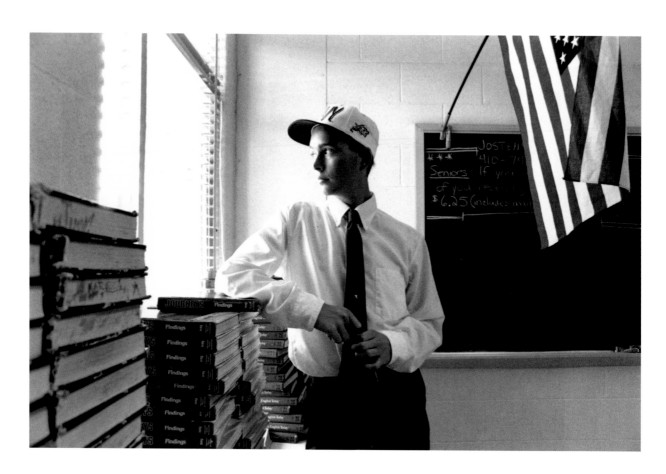

When I started my senior year, I had a new teacher
who said, "One of the rules is 'No hats.'
I can see we already have someone here who doesn't like the rules."
And the whole class jumped up out of their seats,
started screaming at him.

For Heather, the worst part was the hair loss.

Kids can be so cruel.

They would pull her wig off, make fun of her.

PHYLLIS VINES

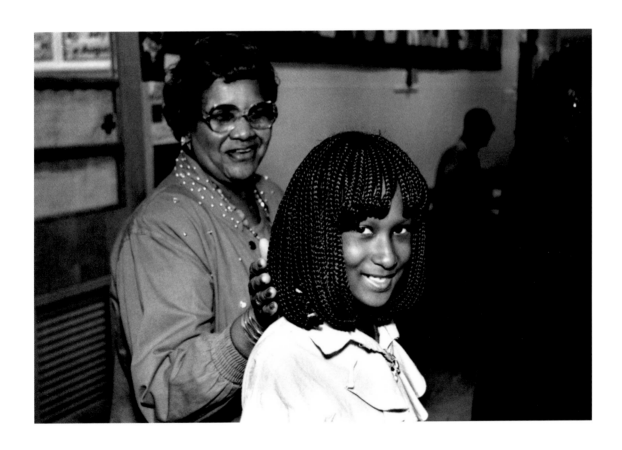

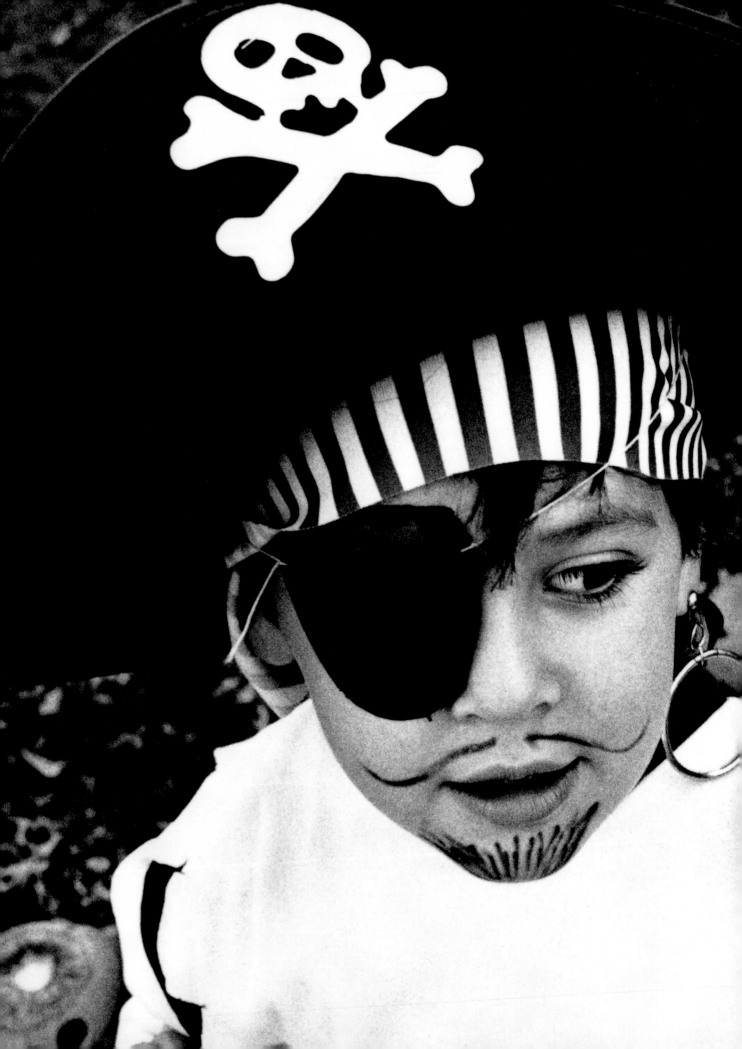

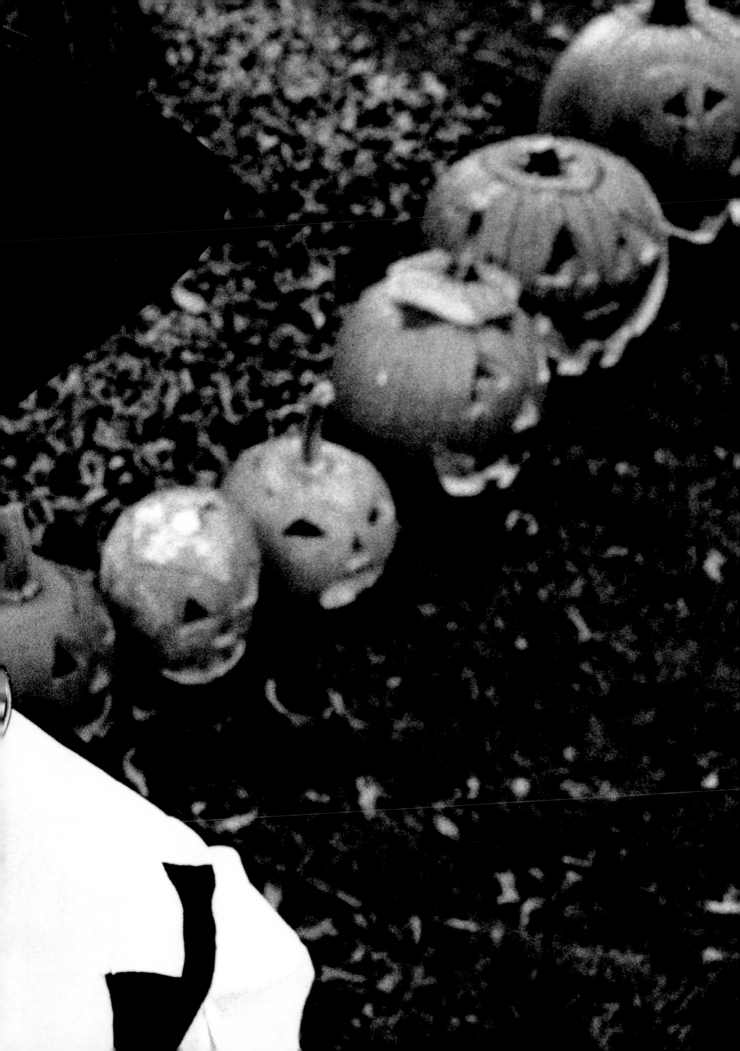

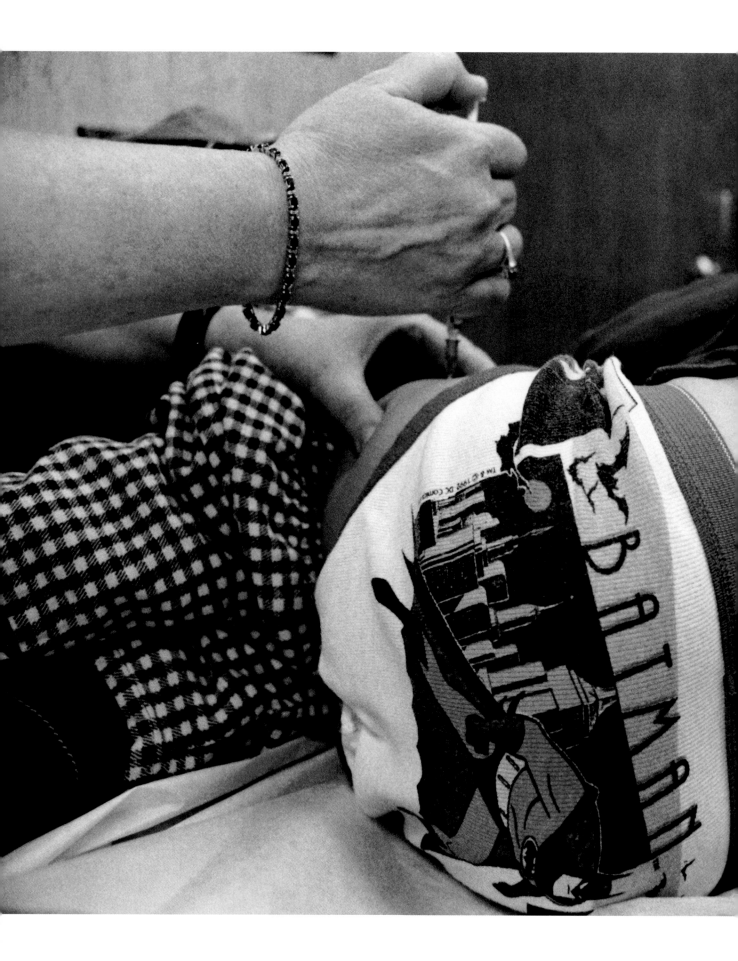

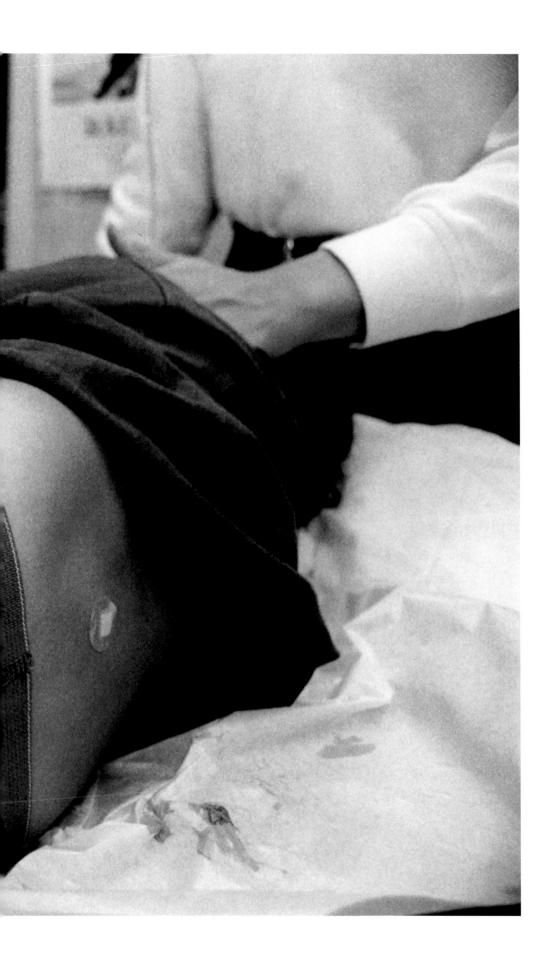

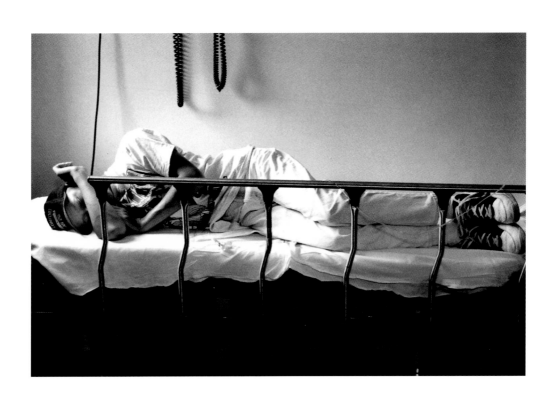

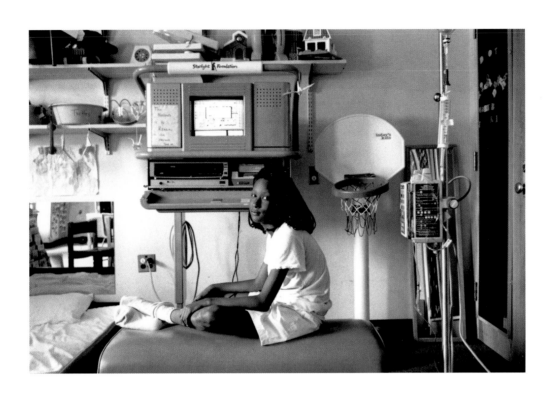

The absolute worst was trying to give him the medicine.

The doctors had this perfect plan,

but I never so lost it as a parent as when I would yell

at Eli to take his medicine.

This was oral yuck, stuff I could barely stand to smell.

The whole concoction...

all I had to do was give him this stuff.

When he said "no" I couldn't do anything.

I couldn't say "You will die if you don't take it."

    Every time he took his medicine,

    he got stickers.

With cancer

you either get better

or you don't.

It doesn't go on forever.

Whoa!

Let me think this was an aberration

but don't tell me it was part of God's plan.

How could you ever believe that?

If you believe that, how could you ever be religious?

Sleeping there was awful.

They tried to help.

I can't imagine leaving him there alone.

I would have a hand on him all night.

I can't imagine not being there.

I felt safer staying in Keith's hospital room.
I could sleep there.
I slept better up there than I could at home.
Nurses had taken over his care.

I'll never forget my first leukemia patient.
When his family heard the diagnosis,
the grandfather got up and tried to throw a chair
through a window.
I was an intern and thought, "This is how you learn."
Last week, that boy sent me
his high school graduation picture. I have it on my wall.

It was a situation I wasn't in control of,
couldn't get control of, didn't know what to do.

Some moments pass too quickly to be photographed.
Sometimes the significant moment is found
in the wink of an eye, the squeeze of a hand, a pinch, a hug, a few words;
the quick movement of a nurse as she swoops up a child
into her arms and heads down the hall;
the brief knowing glances exchanged between two parents.
Some moments are best left to memory, free to come and go.

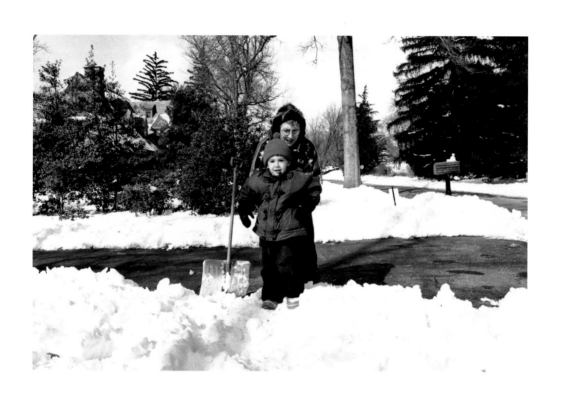

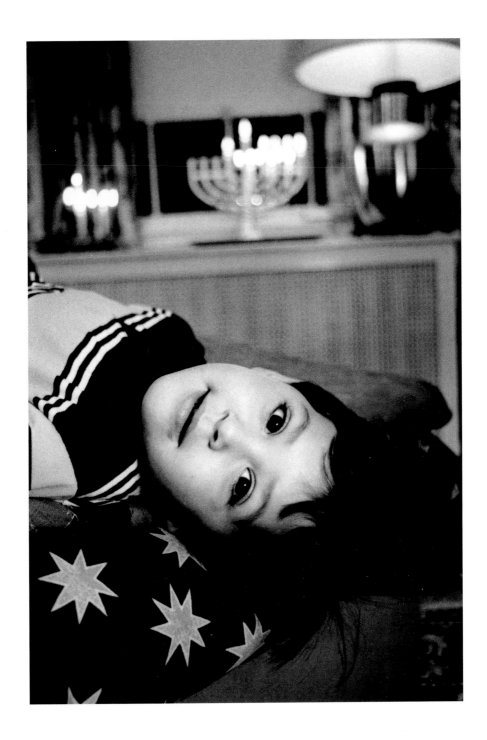

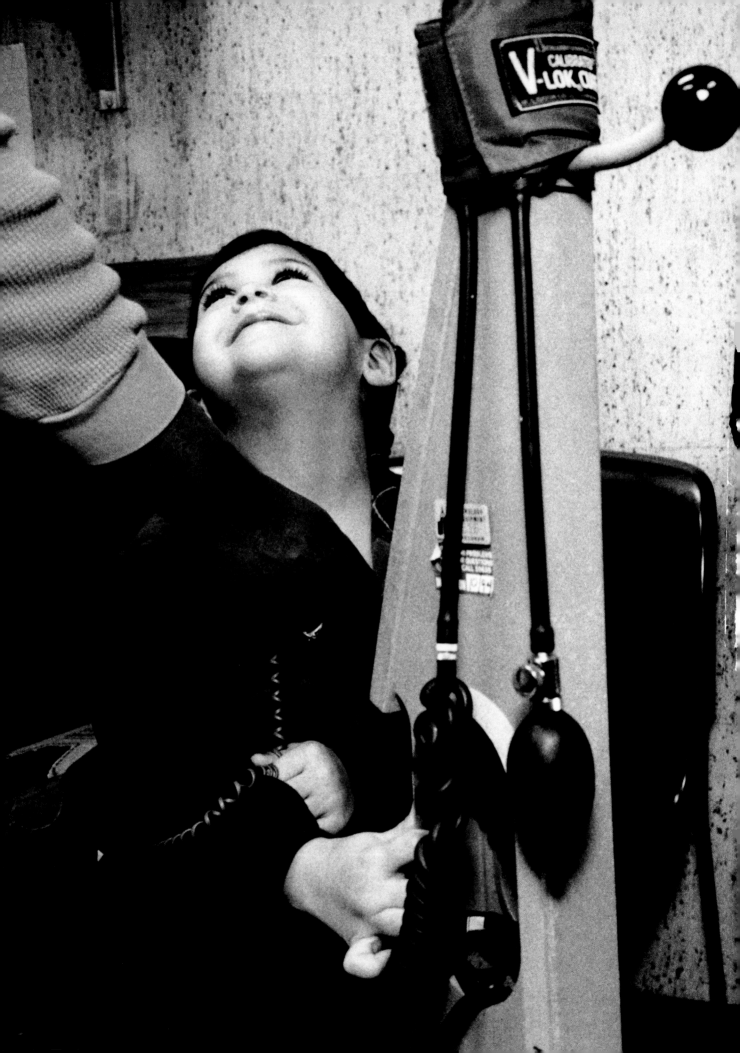

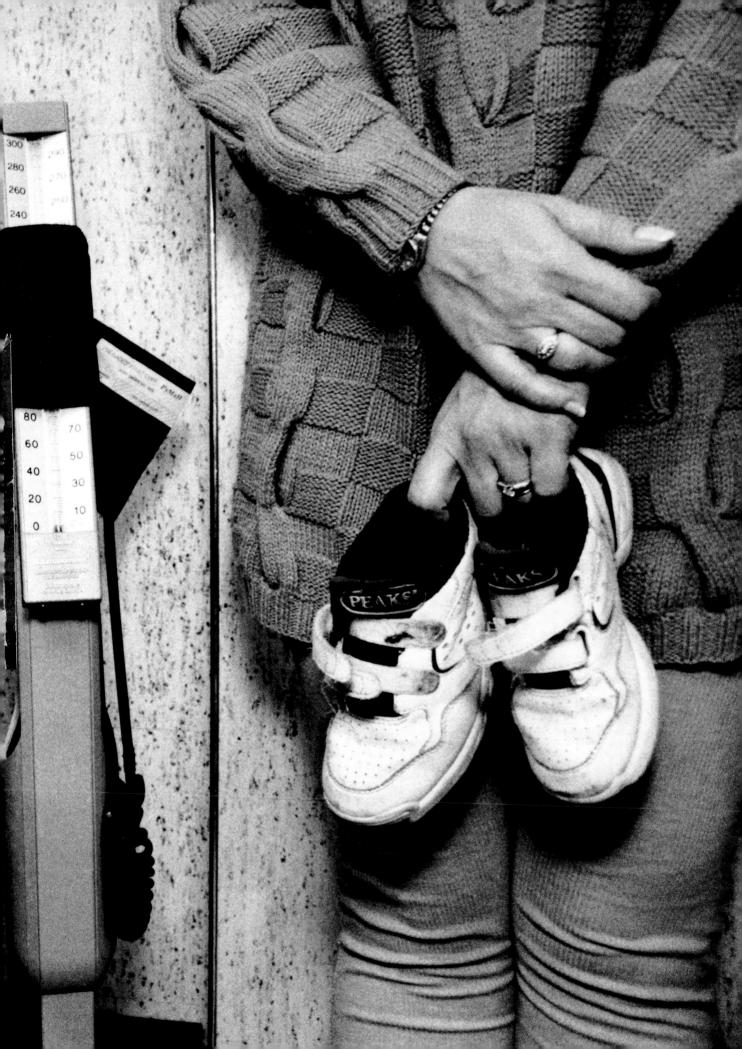

Calm is an illusion. Nothing is at a standstill.
The cancer cells want to have their way even as
the chemotherapy tries to do its job.
These kids are in a constant fight for their lives.

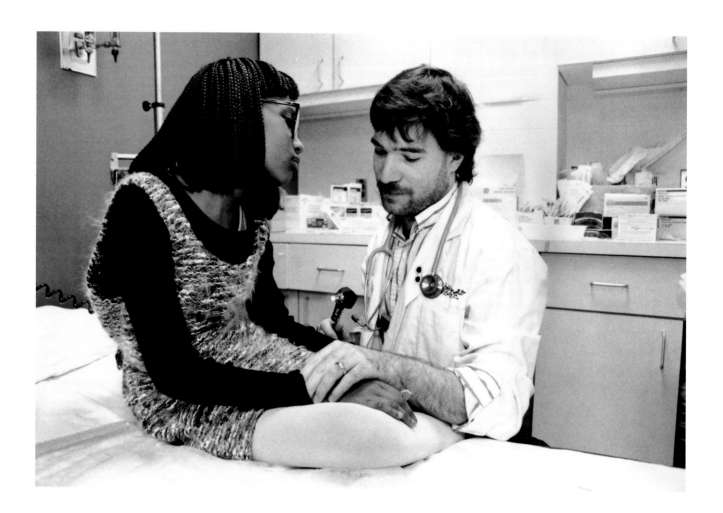

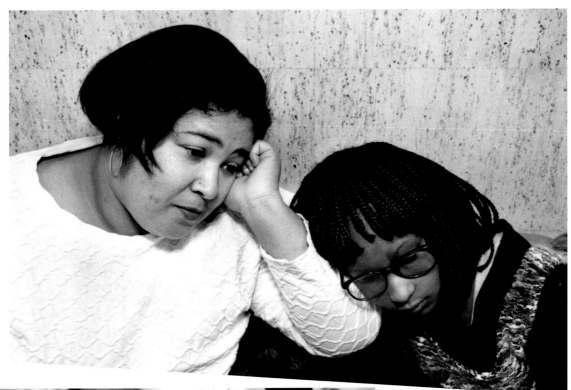

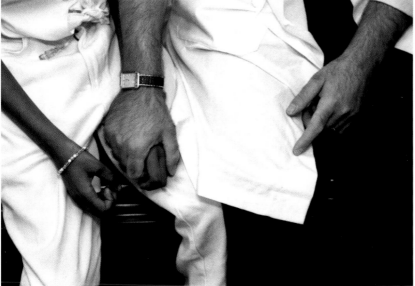

Dr. Goldman fears that Heather's cancer
has returned. With her blood counts too low,
she has developed an infection.

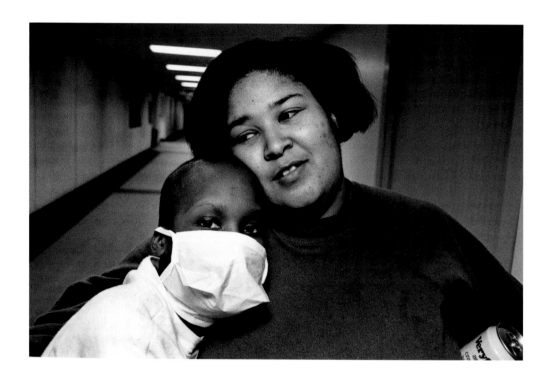

To see if she has relapsed,
a bone marrow analysis is performed.
The procedure goes smoothly
and the marrow is sent to the lab to be prepared
for Dr. Goldman's inspection.
On thin pieces of glass
lies the answer to a very serious question.

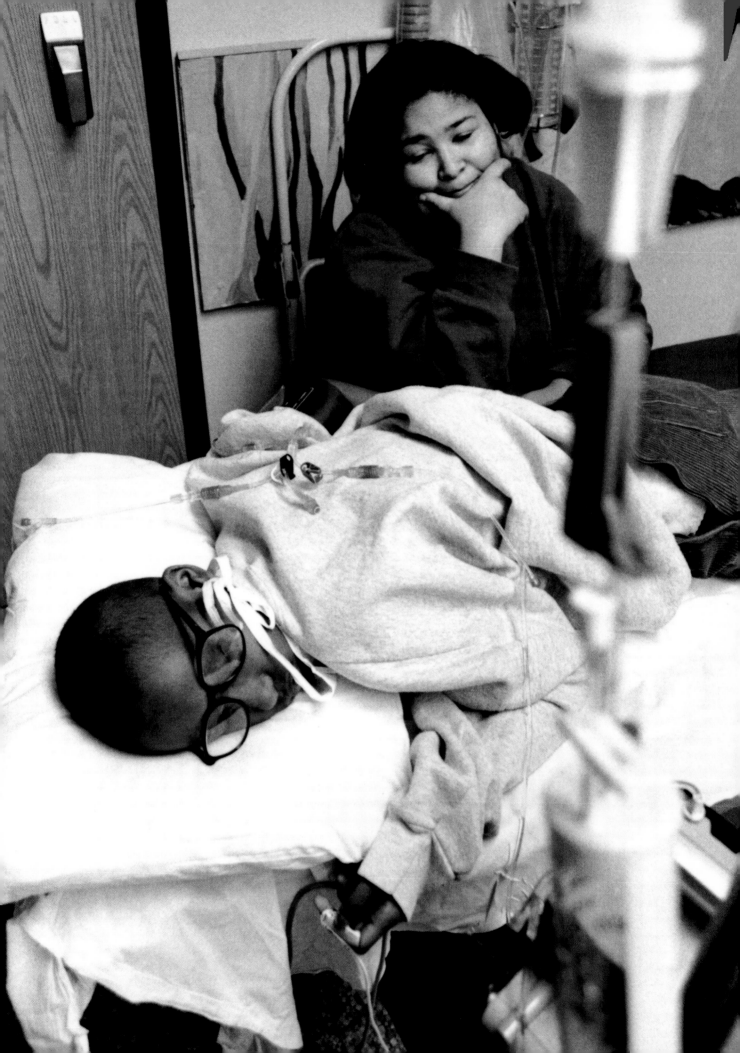

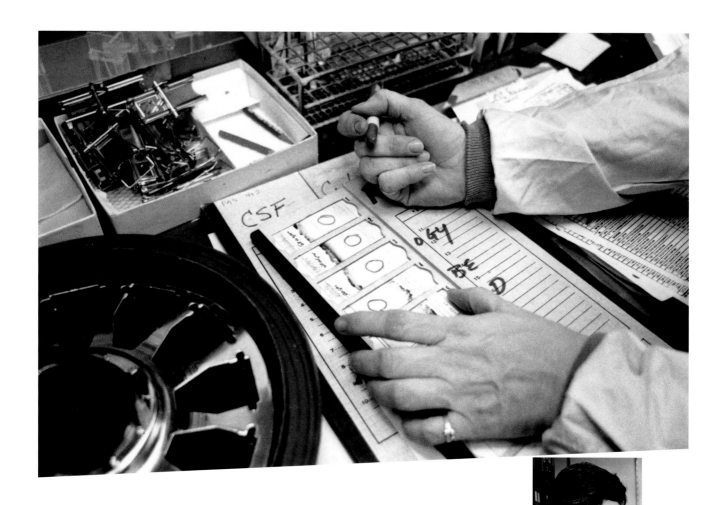

As Dr. Goldman examines the slides,

he finds no evidence of cancer.

Relieved, he hurries to tell Phyllis the good news.

Phyllis has been waiting on 8 East.

As Dr. Goldman approaches, she tries to read his face,

to get the good news a second earlier

or to prepare herself for the worst.

When he tells her everything looks fine,
she smiles broadly, gives him a hug.
Even Heather's nurse breathes a sigh of relief.

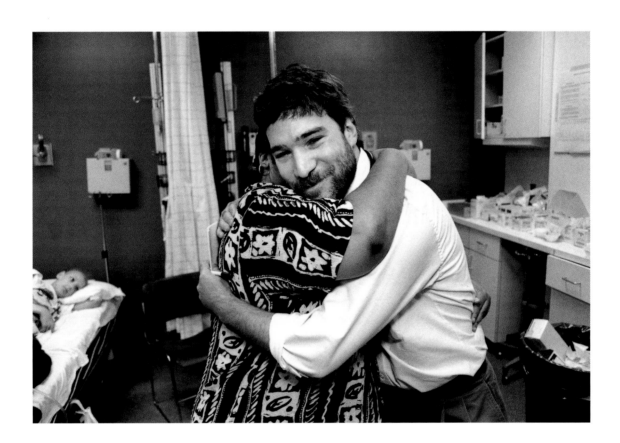

You have to look at the ones who do well,

then you have to think that you helped prolong the good times.

Part of my job is to give them as much good time as possible.

DR. GOLDMAN

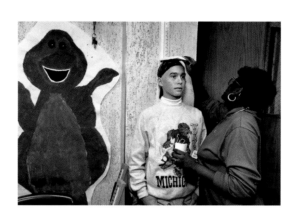

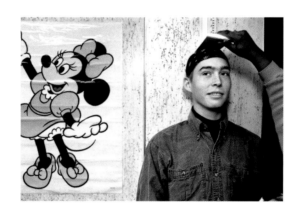

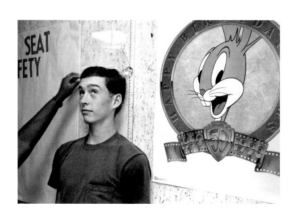

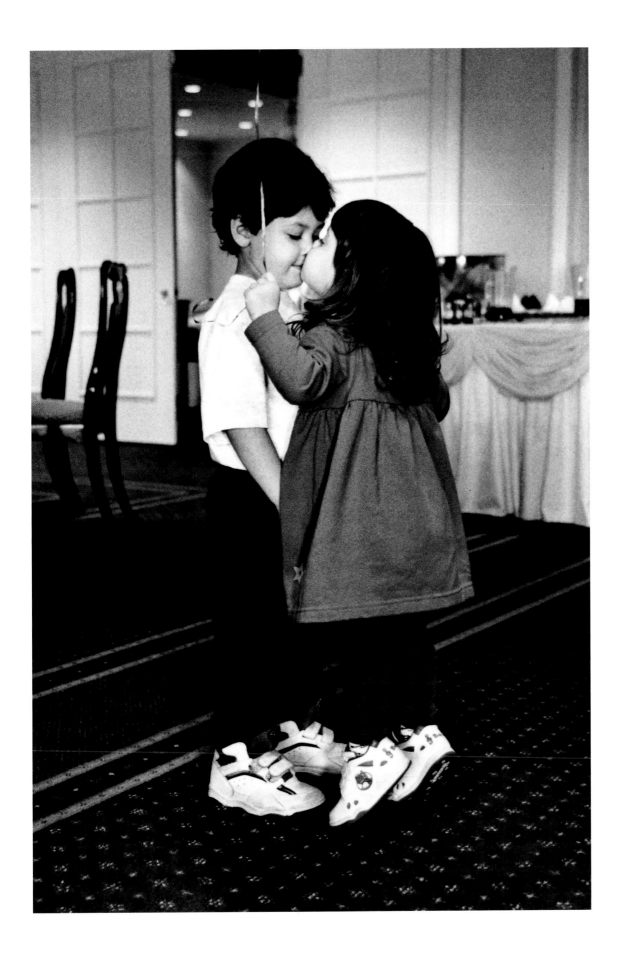

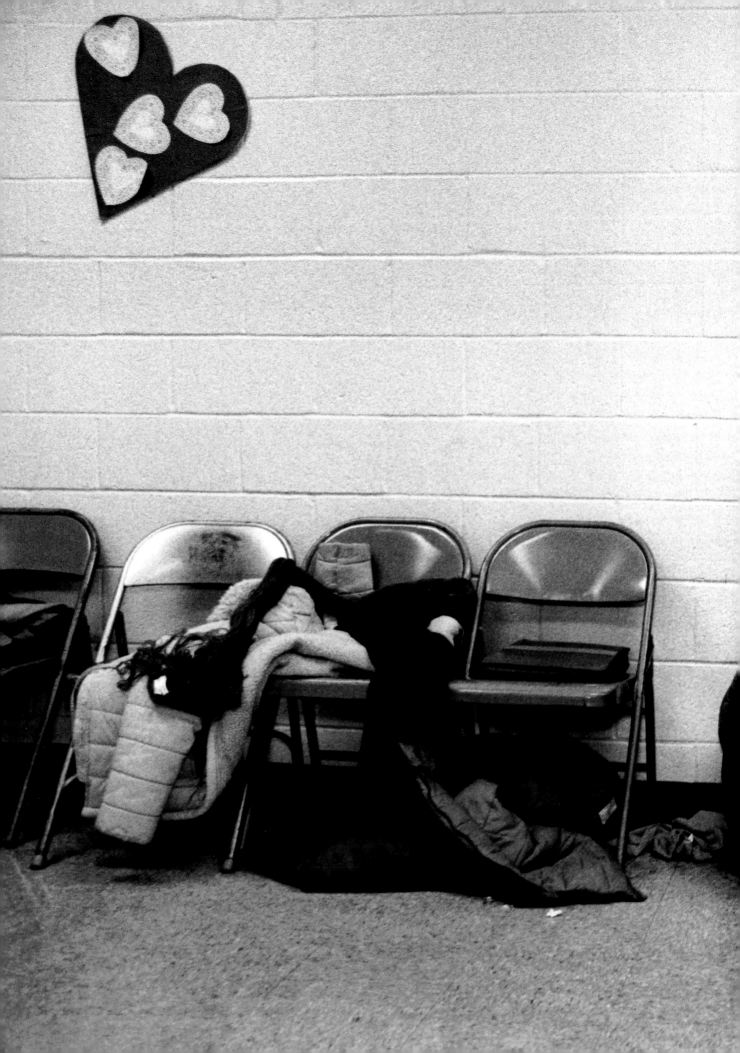

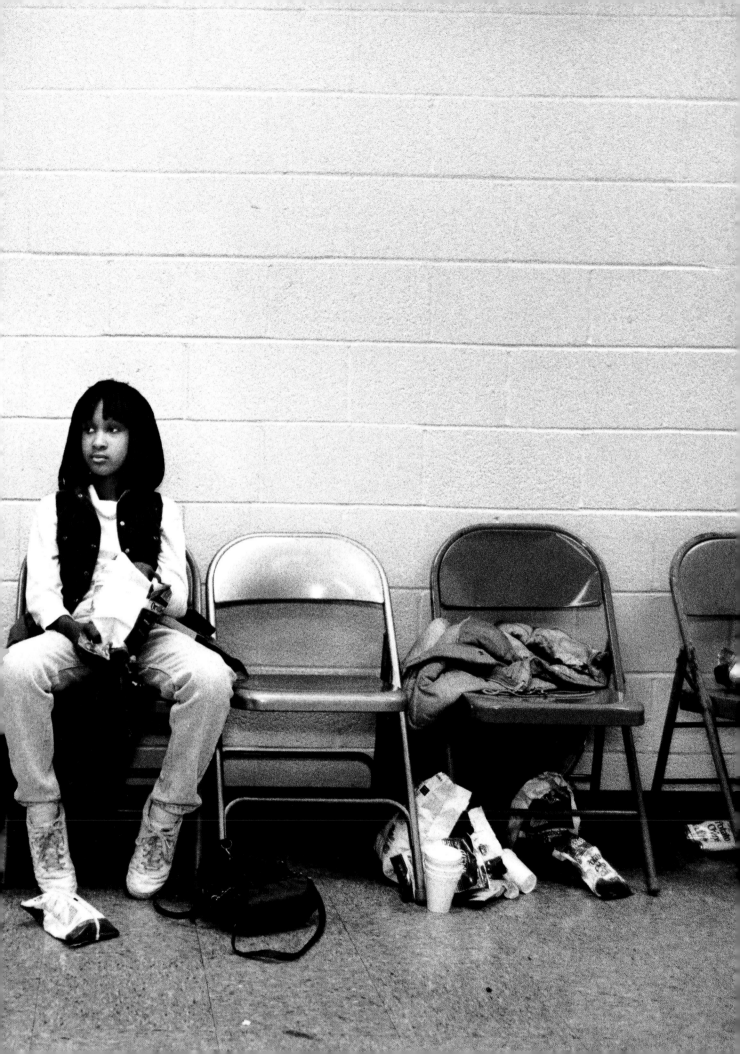

Parents are most nervous when their child comes off therapy.

When therapy stops, their safety net is taken away and they think, "Oh my God!

Now the cancer cells aren't being kept in check anymore."

MADELINE KRIEGER, RN

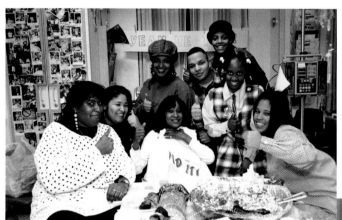

Her prognosis is good.

She's in remission.

She's gotten a fair amount of therapy.

She's got a good chance.

DR. GOLDMAN

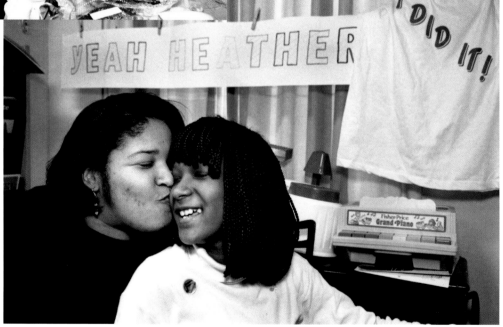

A lot of good has come from this. It brought us closer, it made us a family again.

People prayed and that helped, but it came down to us. We helped each other.

PHYLLIS

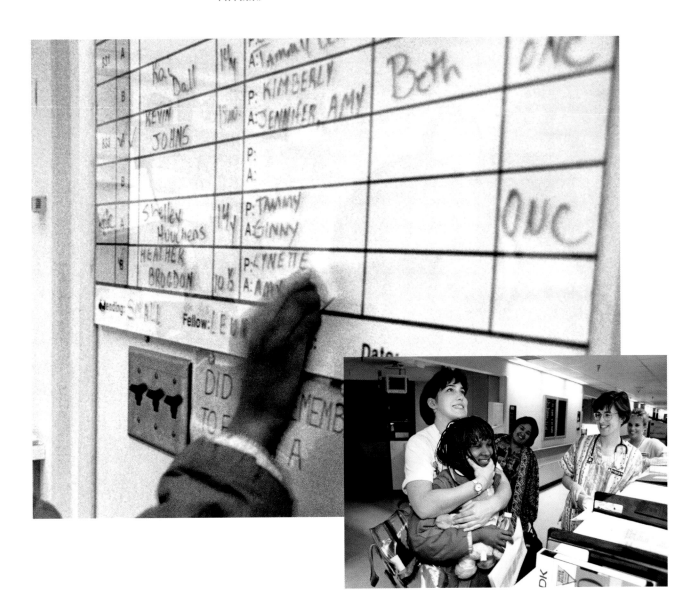

Heather's "end of chemo" party is the party to end all "end of chemo" parties.

Two days later, Heather calls out over the intercom,

"Infusion complete. Time for me to go home!" Tonight, she is happy, cocky, spoiled.

It's late when Heather walks out of her room.

The other children are asleep.

The nursing staff hugs her, tells her to come back and "just visit."

With luck, she will never again be a patient here.

Using an alcohol pad, Heather wipes her name off the 8 East board.

Then it's time to hurry home. Tomorrow is a school day.

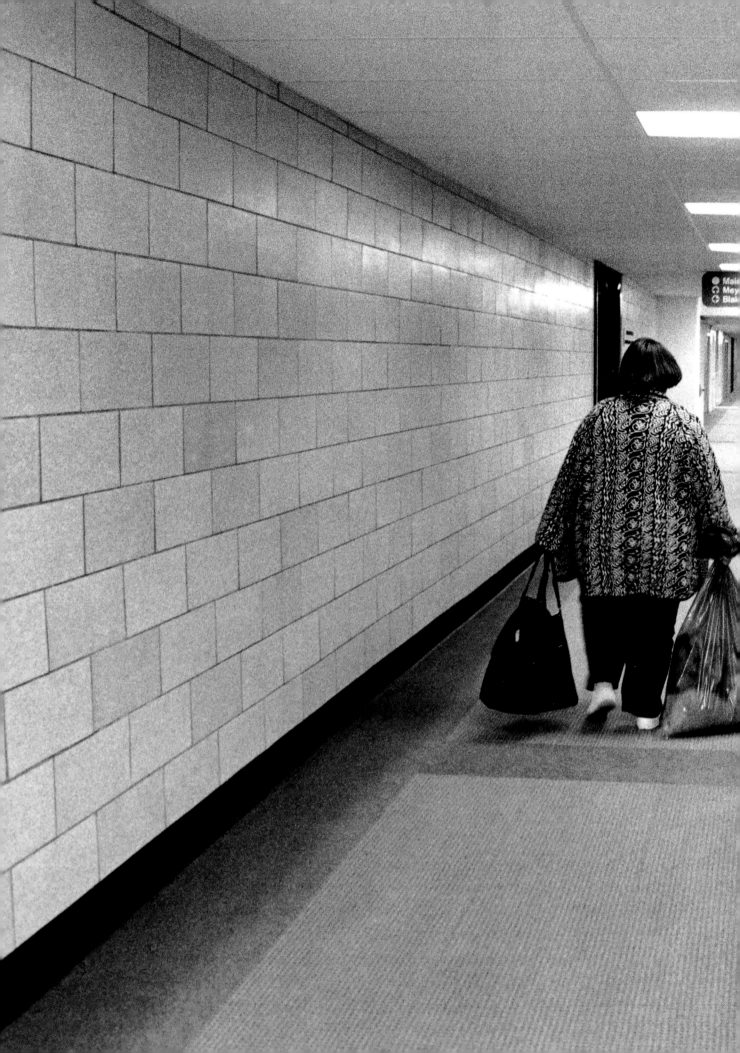

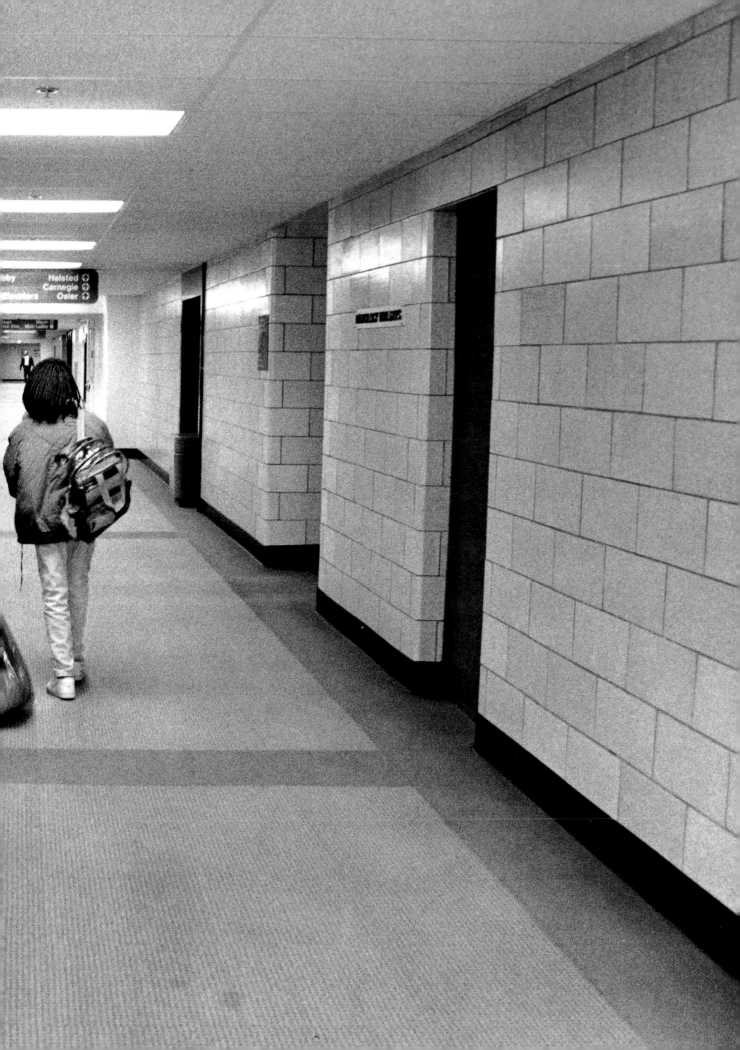

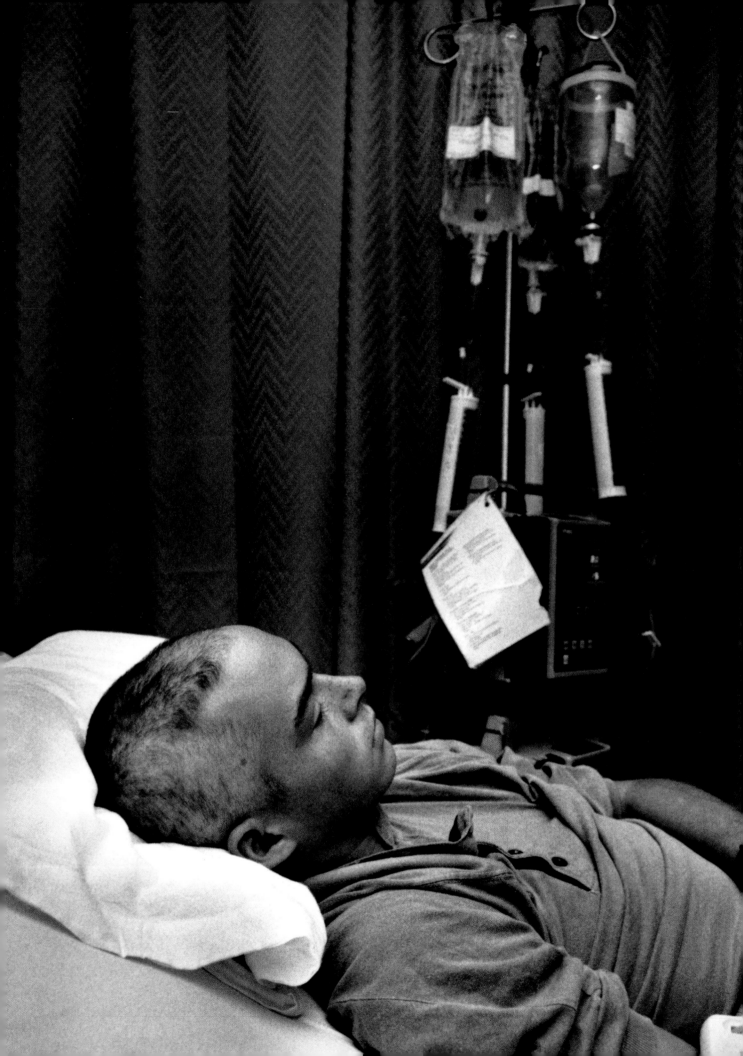

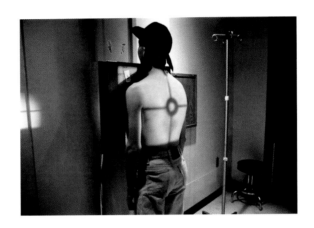

I wasn't afraid of the cancer. The cancer didn't hurt.

It's the chemo that hurts.

I started the chemotherapy because I didn't want to leave my dog.

Who would feed her, look after her?

I did it for Mom and Dad. I didn't do it for me.

I didn't want to do it. Period.

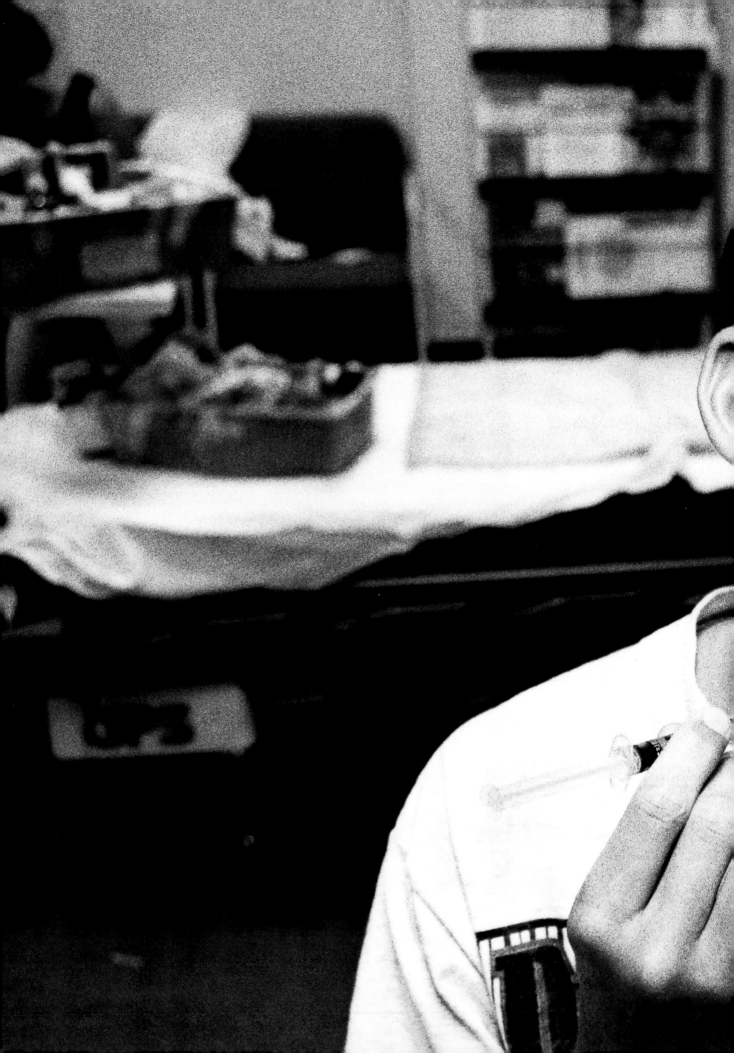

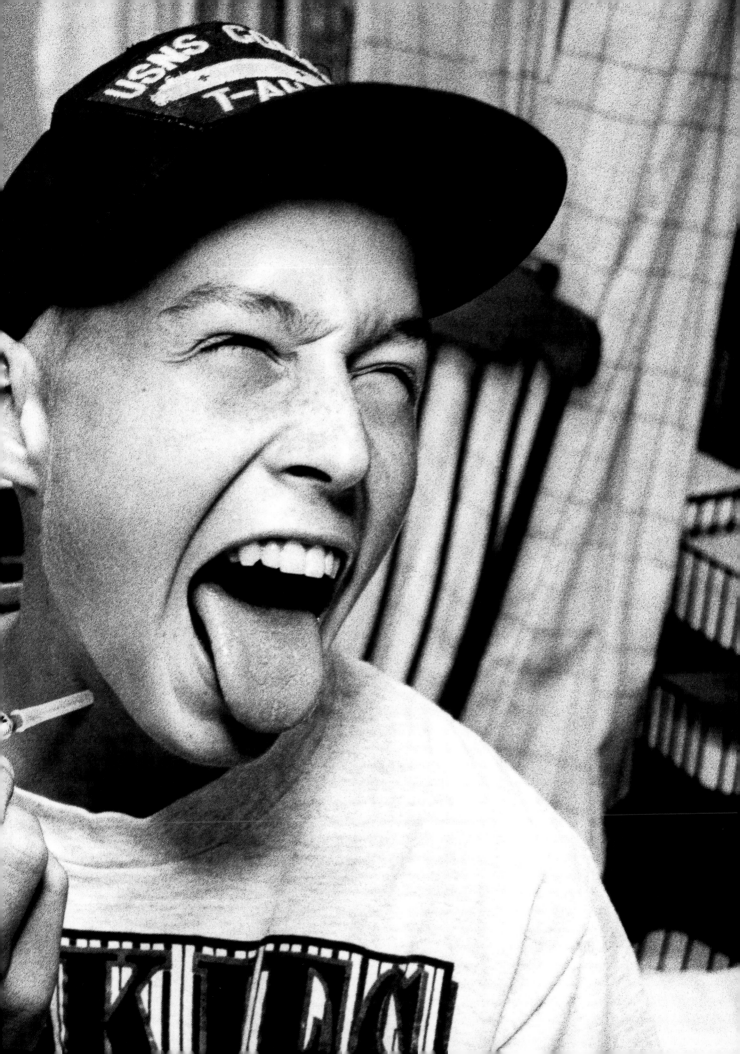

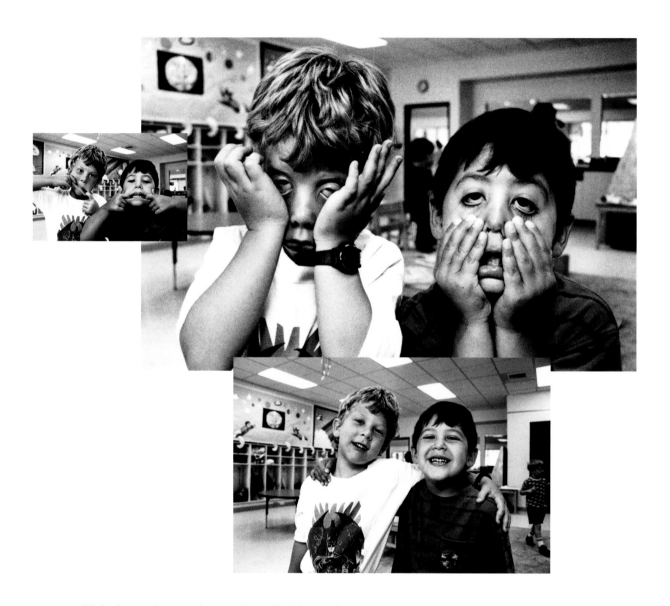

Eli had no real anger about a thing called "cancer."

No "Why Me?"

He didn't realize that he was different.

MARLENE

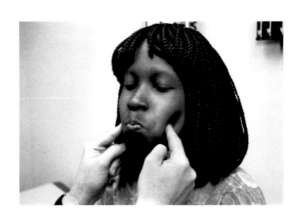

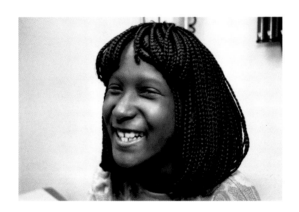

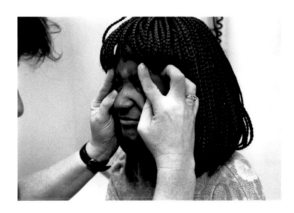

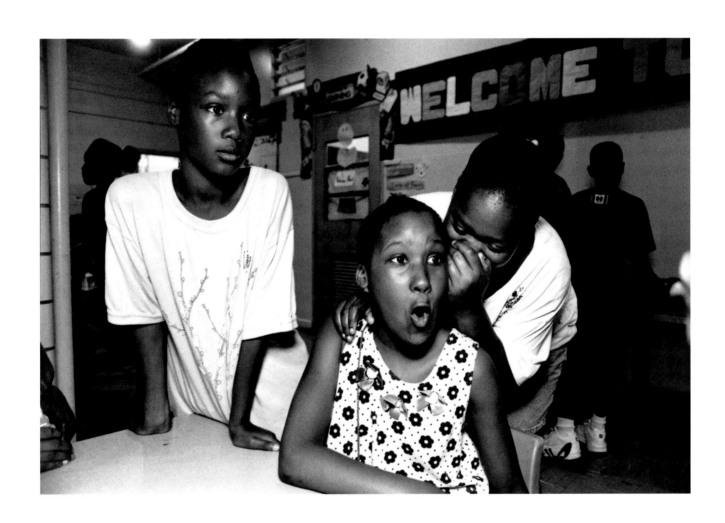

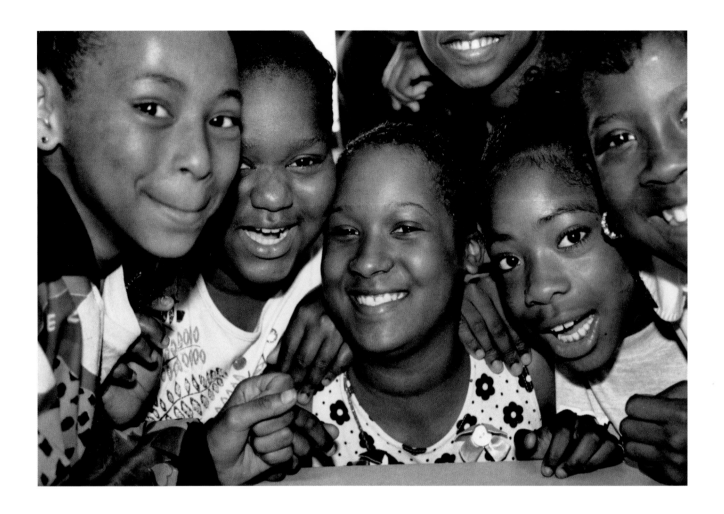

Be a fighter, don't let anyone put you down.

Don't let the disease beat you.

You are still the same person on the inside, before the leukemia.

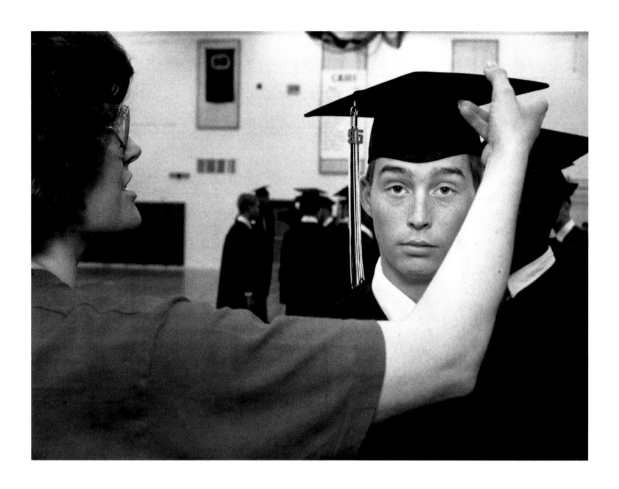

Keith and the graduating class wait in the school cafeteria wearing cap and gown,
joking around, getting excited.
One by one, they enter the auditorium to applause and the flashes of many cameras.
After the invocation and a class poem, it's time for the class song:
"We Are the Champions" combined with "We Will Rock You."
It is sung in an earnest, sentimental, and slightly self-conscious way that suits high school seniors.
Diplomas are awarded and Keith receives his without fanfare.
In the ensuing celebration, he is nowhere to be found.
Cancer has weakened his ties to school and classmates.
No standing around for family pictures, no talking to fellow graduates, no time for reminiscing.
He finished school on time and with good grades. College begins in the fall.

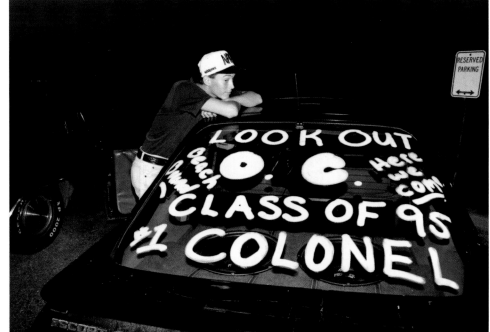

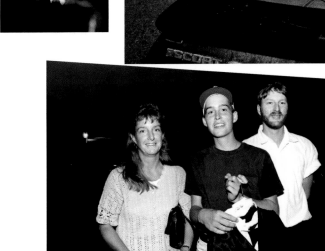

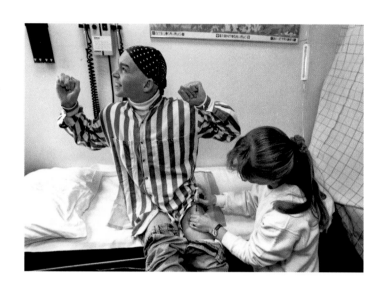

It's like a rollercoaster.

There will be ups and downs.

Hold on.

Sooner or later, hopefully, you'll get off.

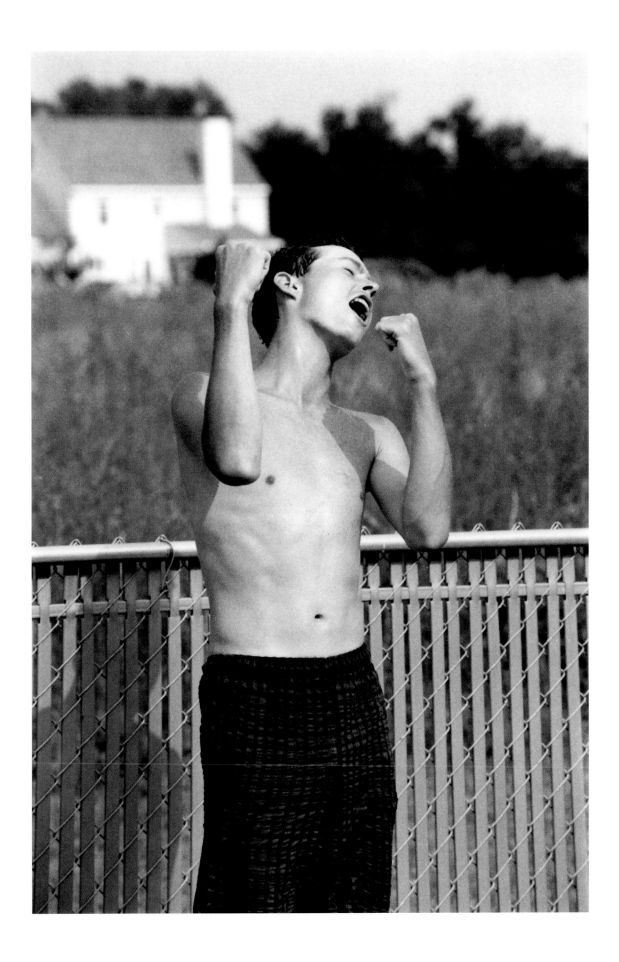

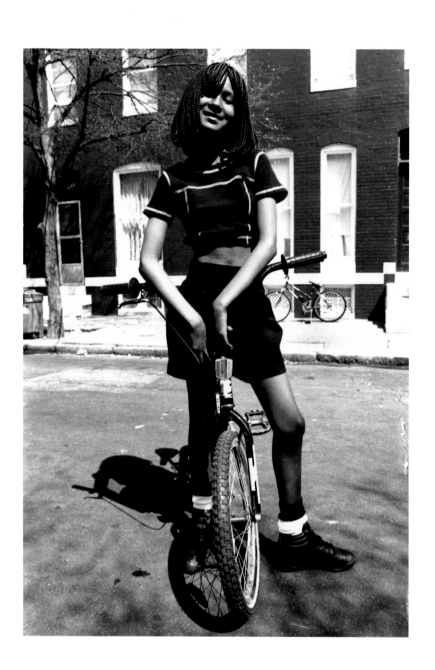
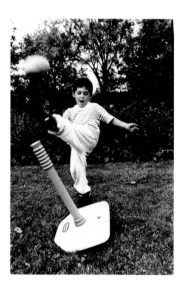

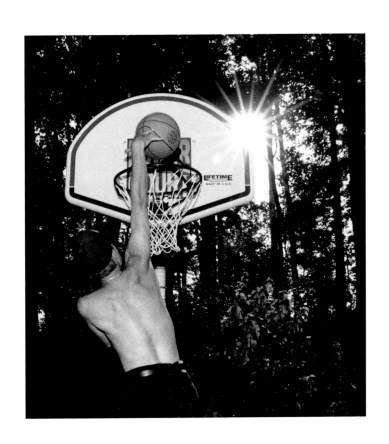

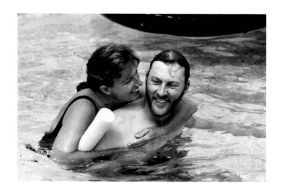

Your friends don't know what to say to you.

Everyone treats you different.

My whole world changed.

It changed my relationship with my other boy.

Dawn and my relationship changed a whole lot.

It will never be like it was before.

Keith's cancer changed the way you feel and think about every situation.

BOB PATRICK

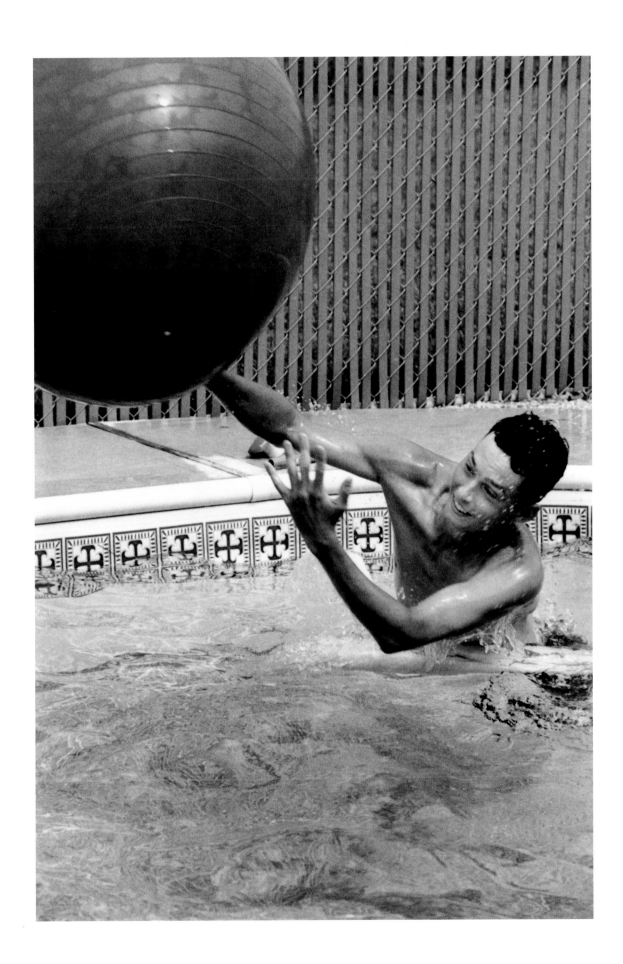

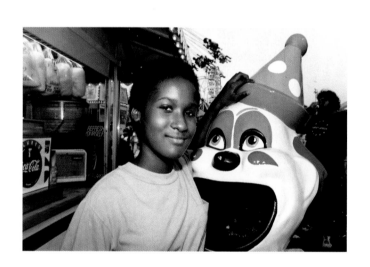

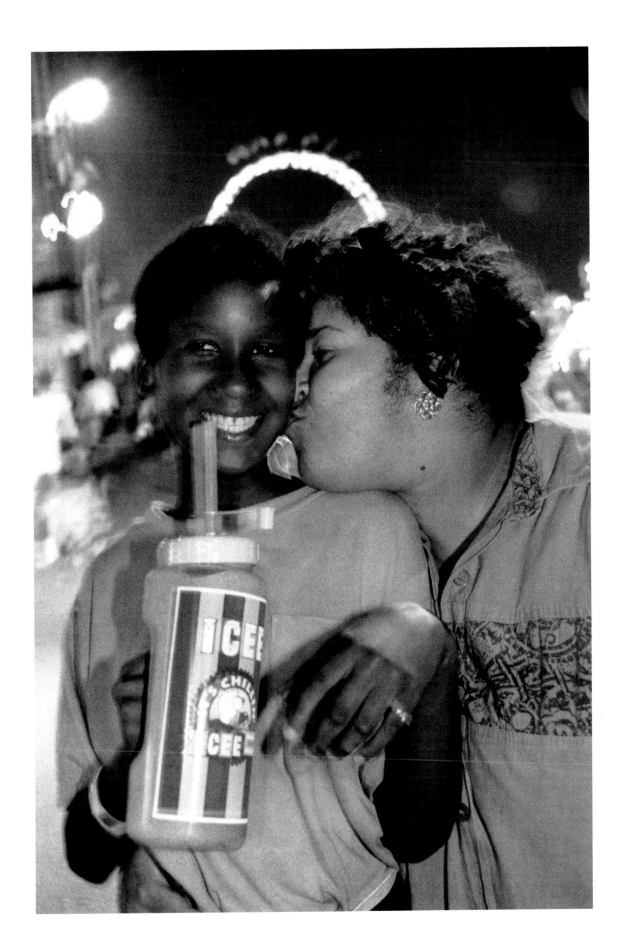

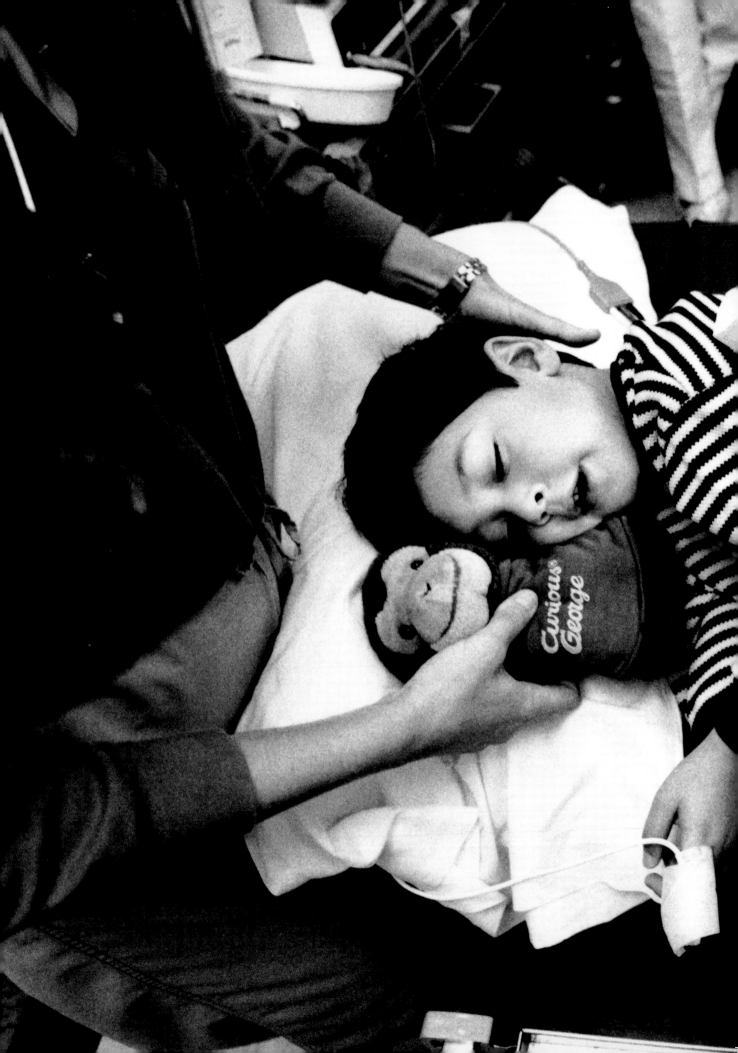

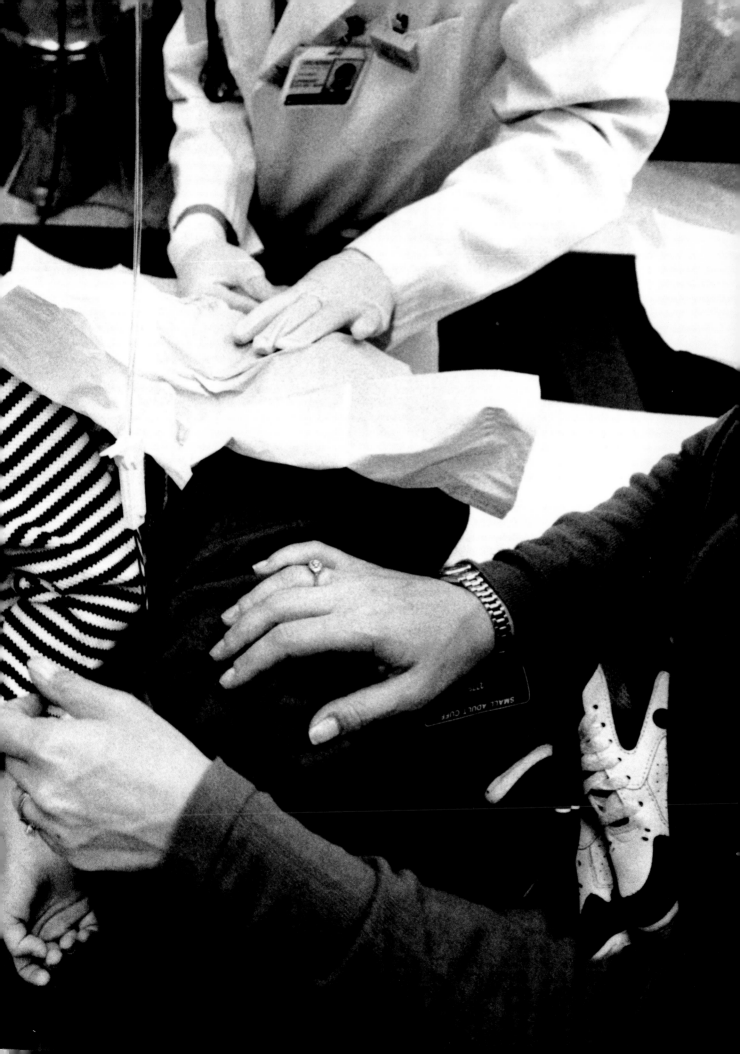

At the start there are about a trillion cancer cells.
Remission means that the number is reduced
to less than a billion. It takes two more years to get rid
of the final billion cancer cells.

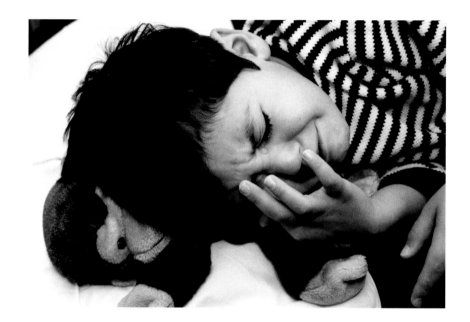

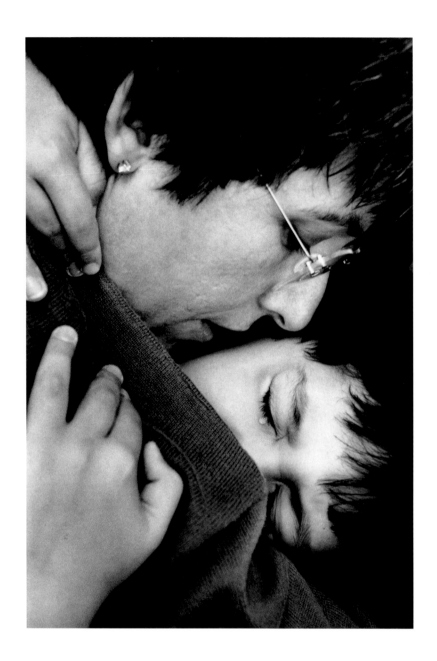

Even when things are going well, the fight against cancer is hard.

After a spinal tap, Eli begins to cry.

His parents are leaving for Miami today and Eli is missing them already.

Marlene hugs him, wipes away the tears, blows his nose, and talks to him.

She tells him how nice she feels to be so missed.

Soon, Eli is getting a soda, a prize from the toy chest, and heading home for lunch.

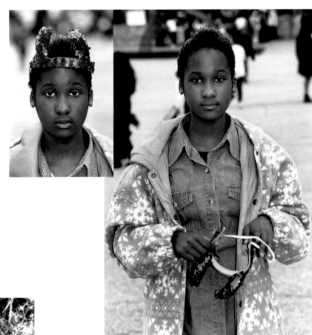

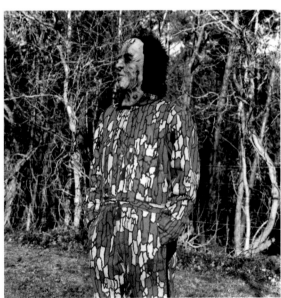

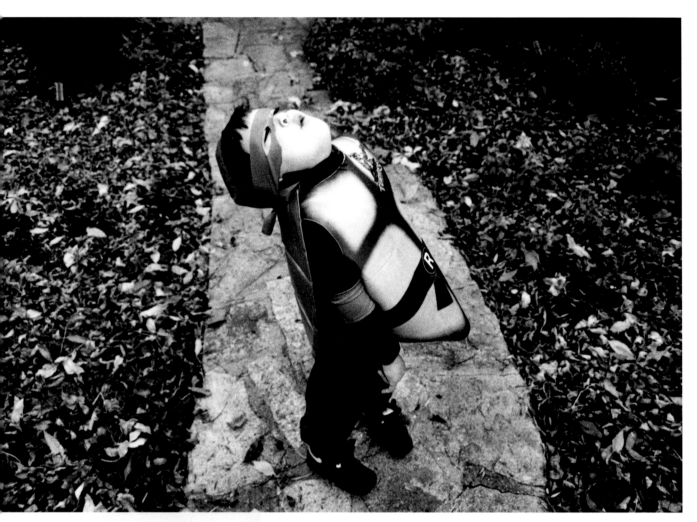
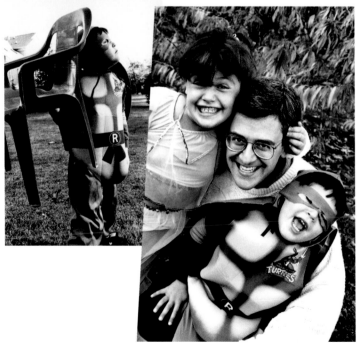

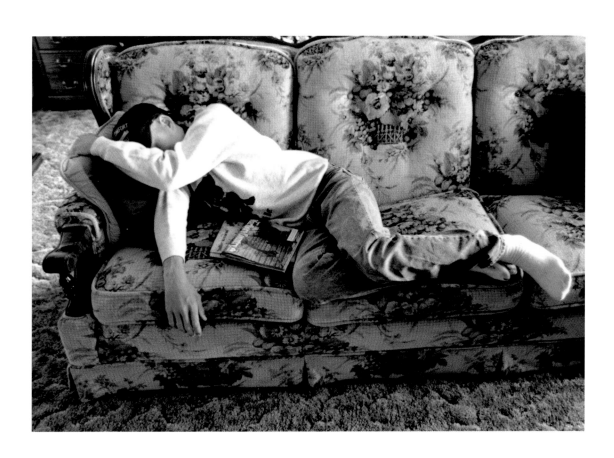

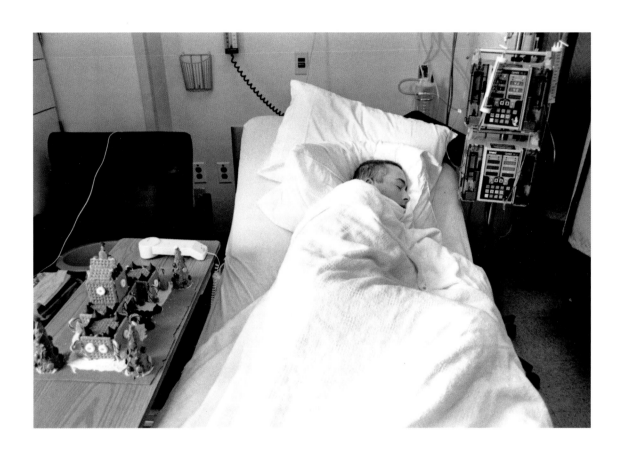

The only times I went down to the playroom was to play Nintendo

and to make a gingerbread house.

I had the playroom to myself and was there making it one day—

putting icing on it and licking my fingers.

Then Dr. Kastan walked in and said, "Keith, please don't eat that paste!"

He thought it was glue!

A Hopkins doctor and dumb as a nail.

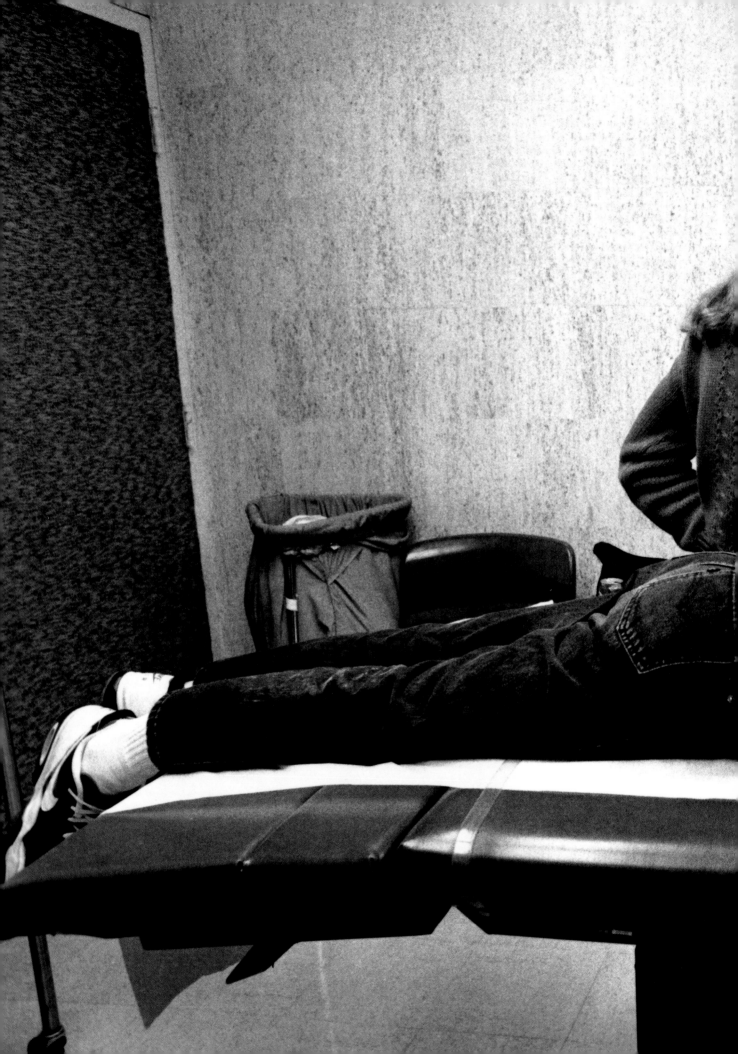

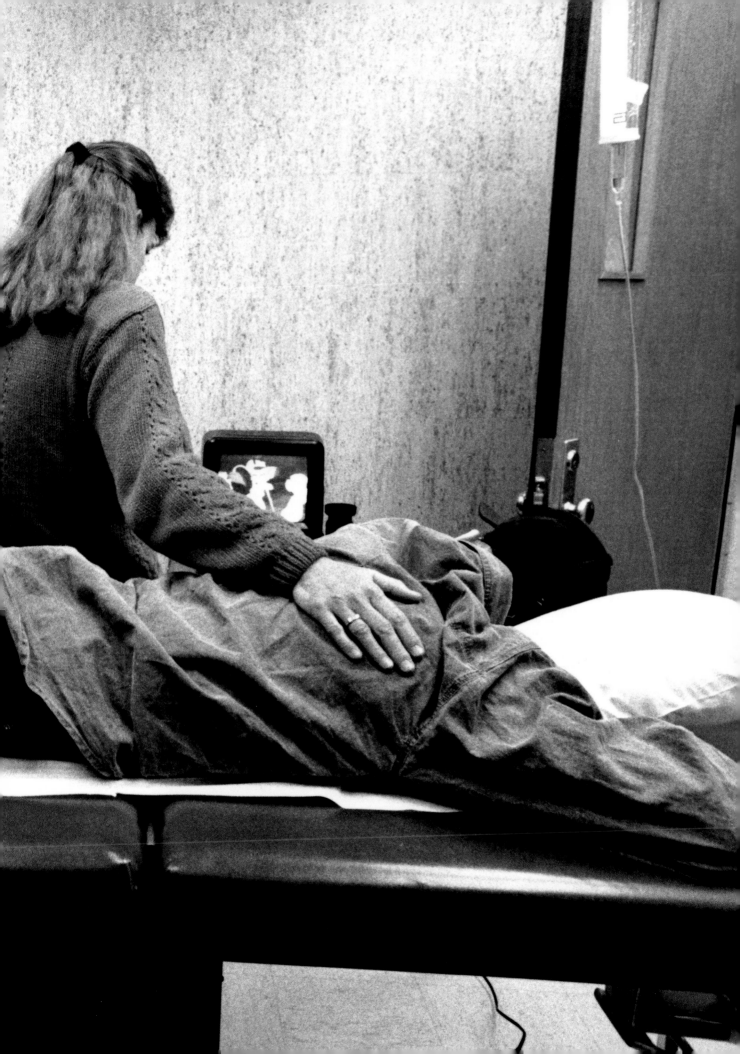

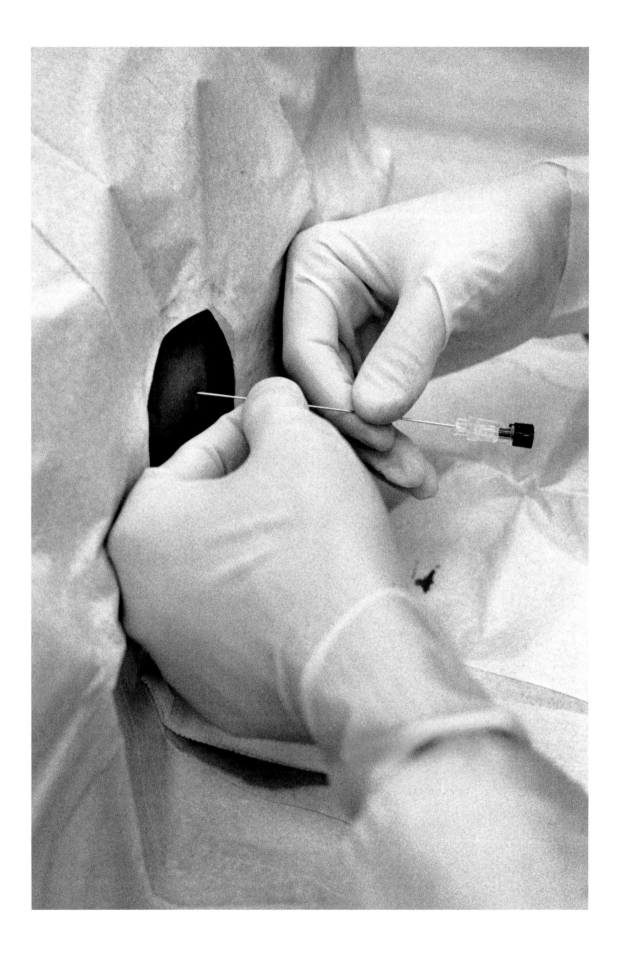

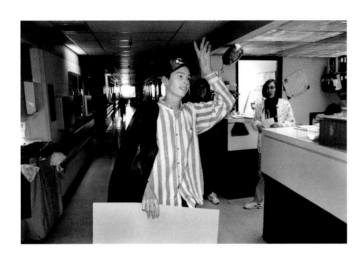

Chemo is maturity in a bottle.
When you have to fight for tomorrow, you grow up today.
You fight better as an adult.
I'm going to be as different as I want to be.
I'll say whatever I want to say.

Keith is a typical teenager.
Keith never believed that something bad would happen to him
and he went on with his life as if nothing had happened.
And that's wonderful.

DR. KASTAN

These are people you'll remember all your life.

TERESA SWEENEY, RN

Now it's Keith's turn to say goodbye to 8 East.
There's no "end of chemo" party, no cake. Keith just wants to go home.

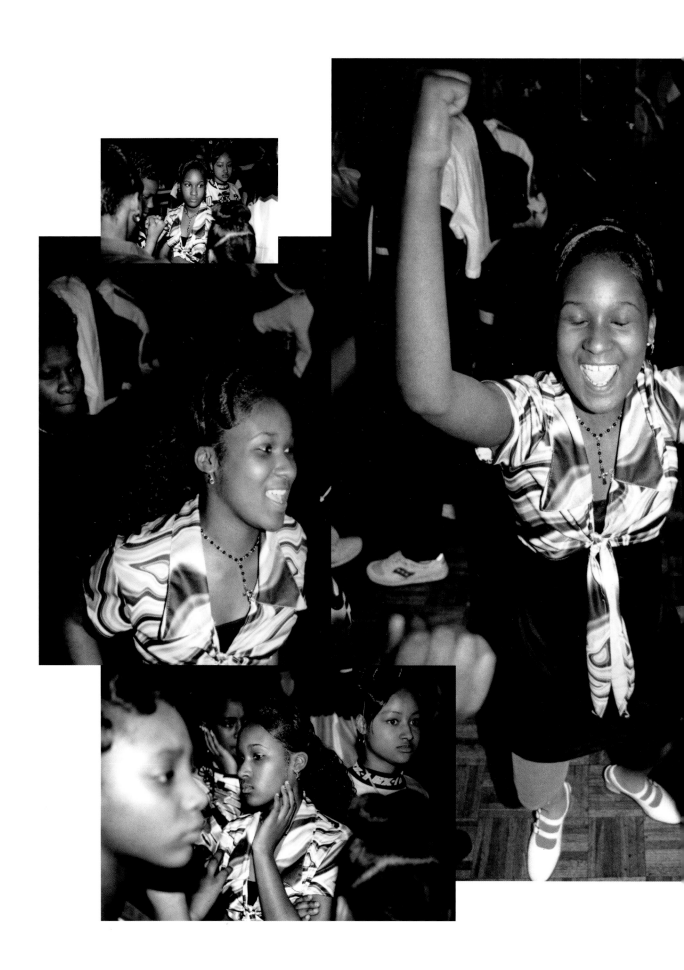

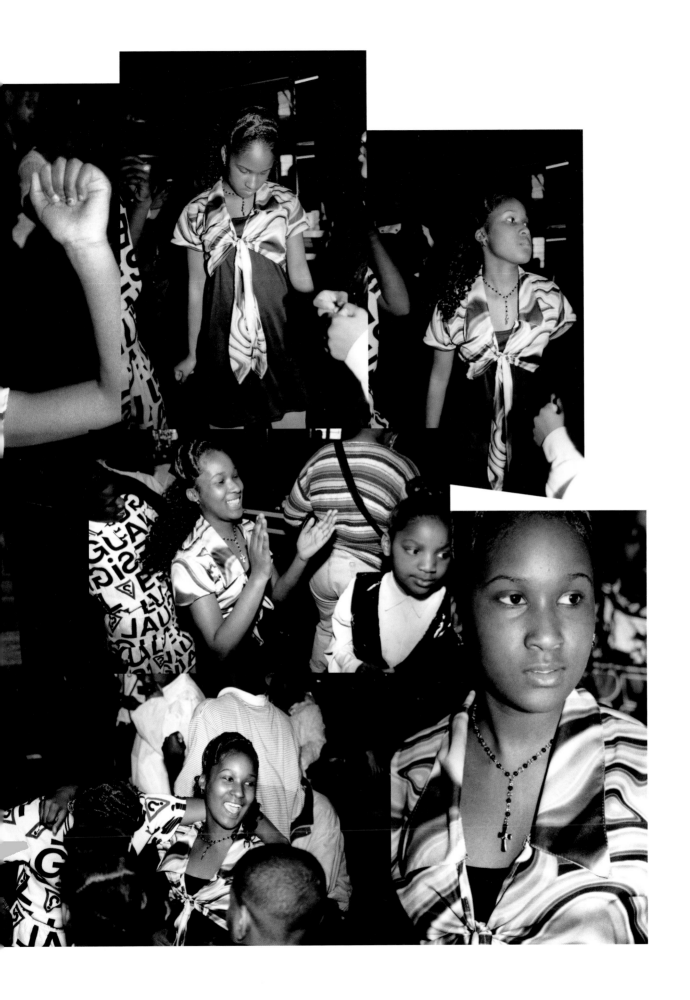

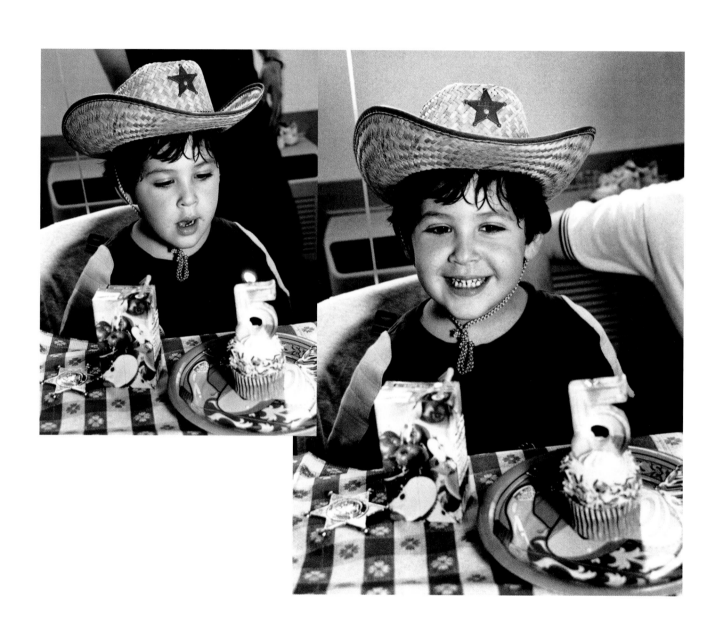

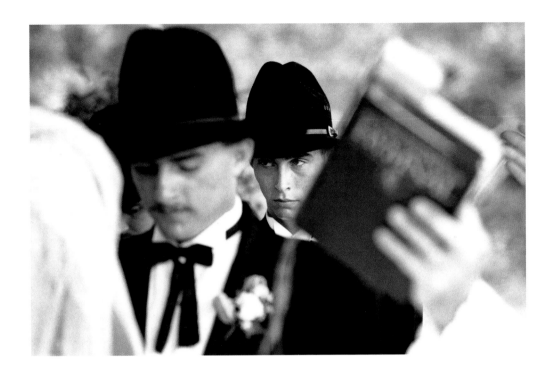

Even now, at his brother's wedding, five months after the end of chemo,

his overnight bag is still packed.

I can't unpack it. Cancer never leaves. It's always a part of your life.

DAWN

The work goes on.
Until every childhood cancer story has a happy ending,
the clinic will be full of movement and noise
as nurses, doctors, and families meet here, share laughter and tears,
and look for a way to save the lives of their children.

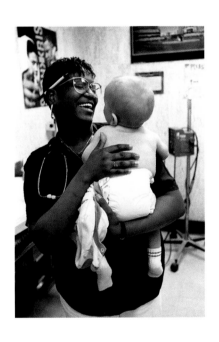

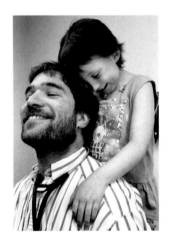

GLENDA CHAPMAN, NST

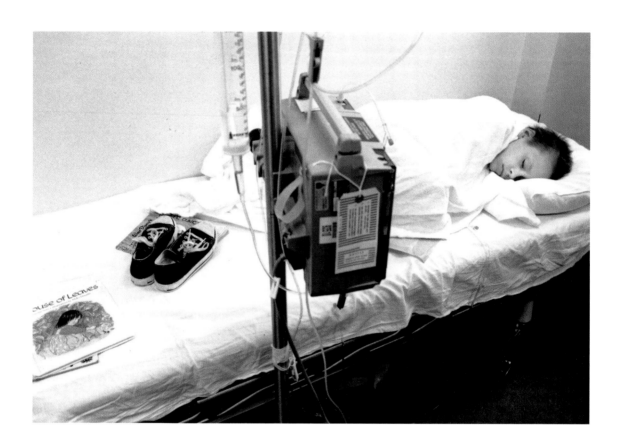

Danny

Michael

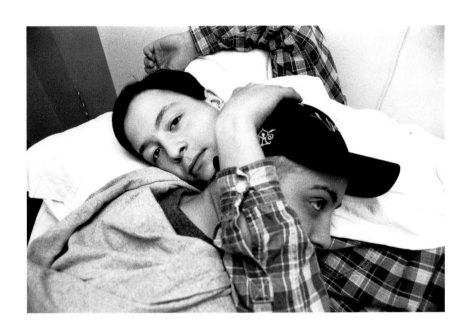

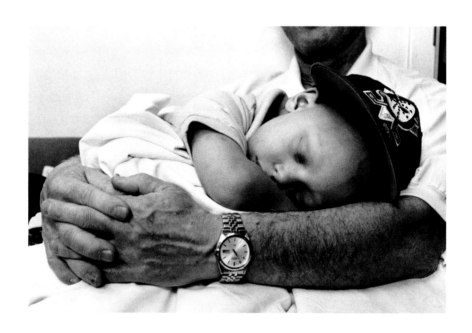

Matt

Lenae

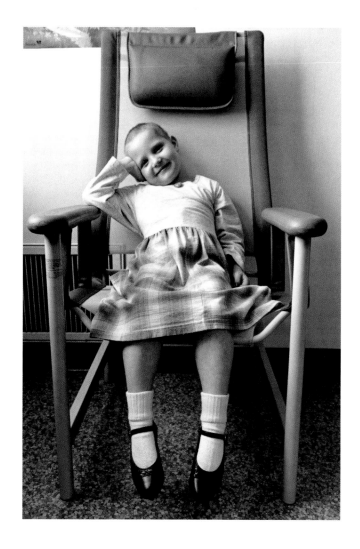

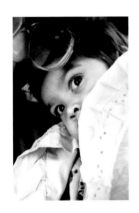

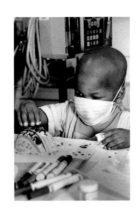

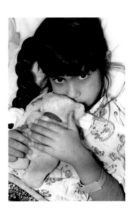

Marie   DeShawn   Rachel

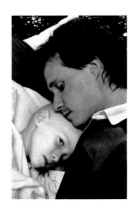

Urijah

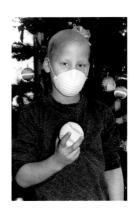

Danny

I photographed
fifty-four children with cancer;
seventeen have died.

The nurses are there year after year.

They see patients from diagnosis through treatment or death or relapse.

They are equipped to help the parents go through all this.

DR. GOLDMAN

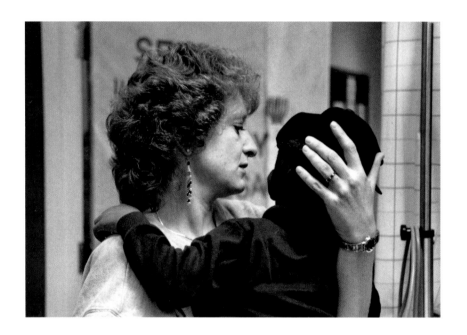

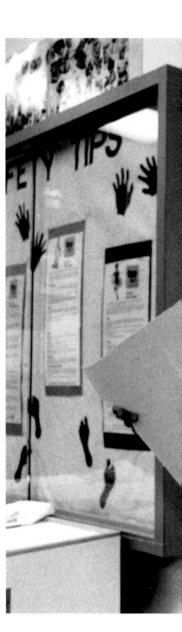

I'm having friends over for pizza and beer,

but the pizza is looking less and less important.

MADELINE KRIEGER, RN

DR. MARIA PELIDIS

You spend a lot of energy helping families.

You become an extended part of their family.

They count on you for a lot...for everything.

SUE RODGERS, RN

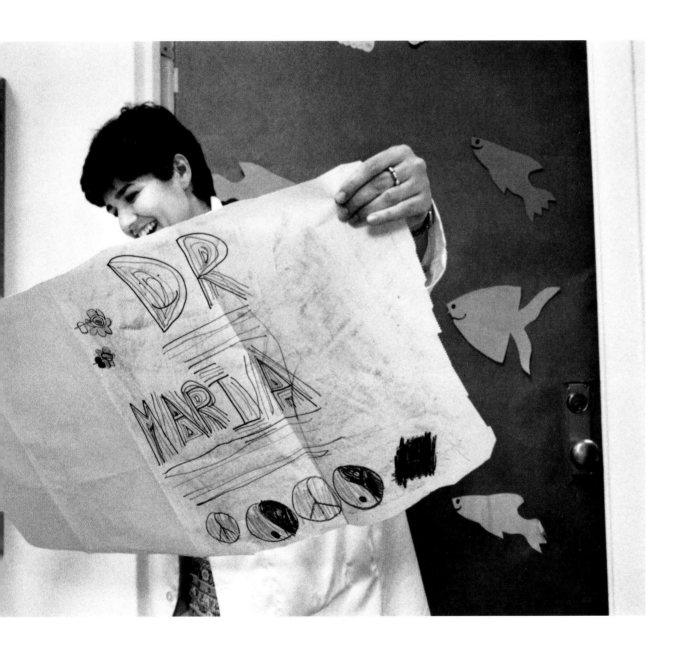

I get angry that we can't cure certain diseases. It drives me in the laboratory.

I have this goal that what we are doing in the laboratory is going to help many more people

than I could help as an individual physician. This work makes me who I am.

DR. KASTAN

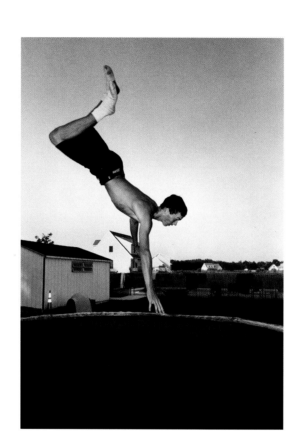

"What are the odds that all three of your kids will make it?"

Soon after I began my work, a nurse asked this question. I had no answer for her. From the beginning, I wondered how these stories might end. I was afraid to think that these kids might die in front of my eyes. There were times when it looked like the worst might come true, that cancer might win.

I look closely at these pictures and see children who were not so lucky—children who died, even as my kids lived.

No one can say with certainty how any fight with cancer will go. When I told Keith that my photography was nearly done, that I could soon tell his story, he smiled and said,

"For me, the story is never over."

He's right. No one can guarantee that Eli, Heather, and Keith won't relapse. There won't be a day when a doctor will say: "It's gone. It won't be back. No need to worry."

But today, there is no sign of their cancer. For every day they remain in remission, their future grows brighter.

When will everyone stop knocking on wood? Will life ever return to normal? I'm looking forward to the day when their cancer is no longer a threat, nearly forgotten. I'm looking forward to Eli's bar mitzvah, Heather's high school graduation, Keith's wedding.

They have spent too much of their young lives fighting cancer. Still, they celebrated birthdays, attended school, fought with siblings, made new friends, got into trouble. They remained kids.

For me, these journeys through cancer were about more than a disease; they were about childhood itself, the fleeting time of three young people filled with more heartache and joy than most.

Eli, Heather, and Keith, free from the struggles of these years, are moving ahead, discovering what else life has in store for them.

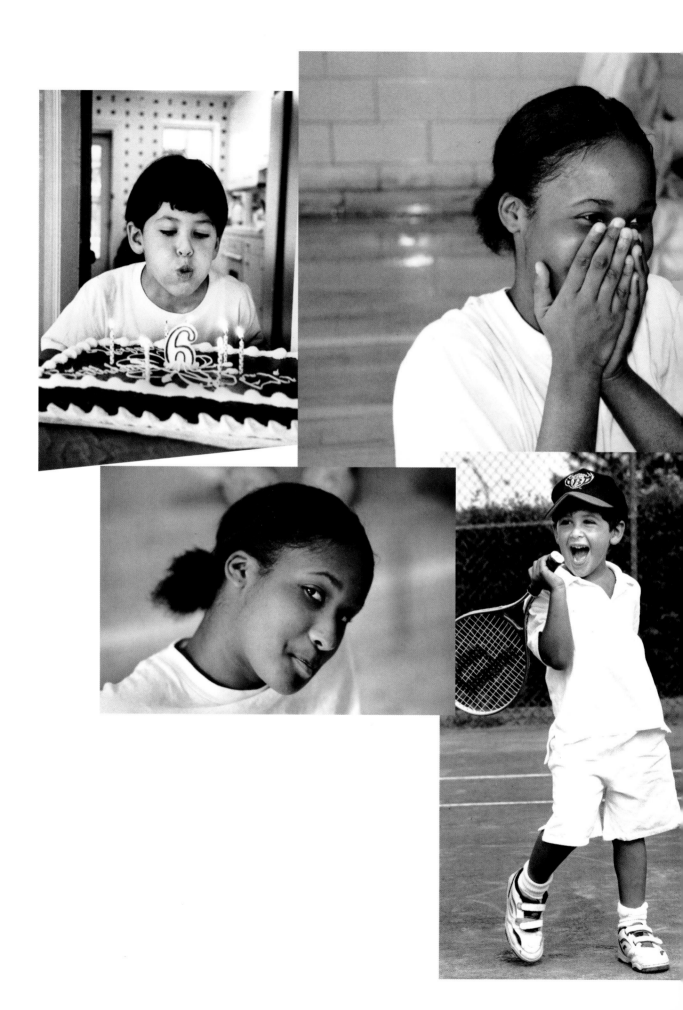

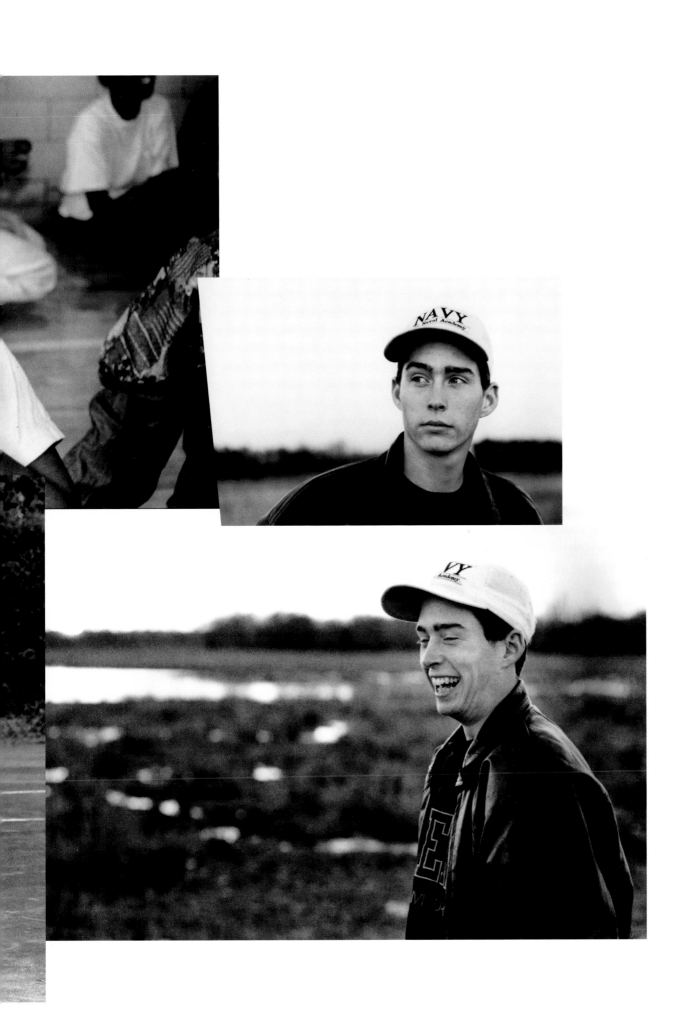

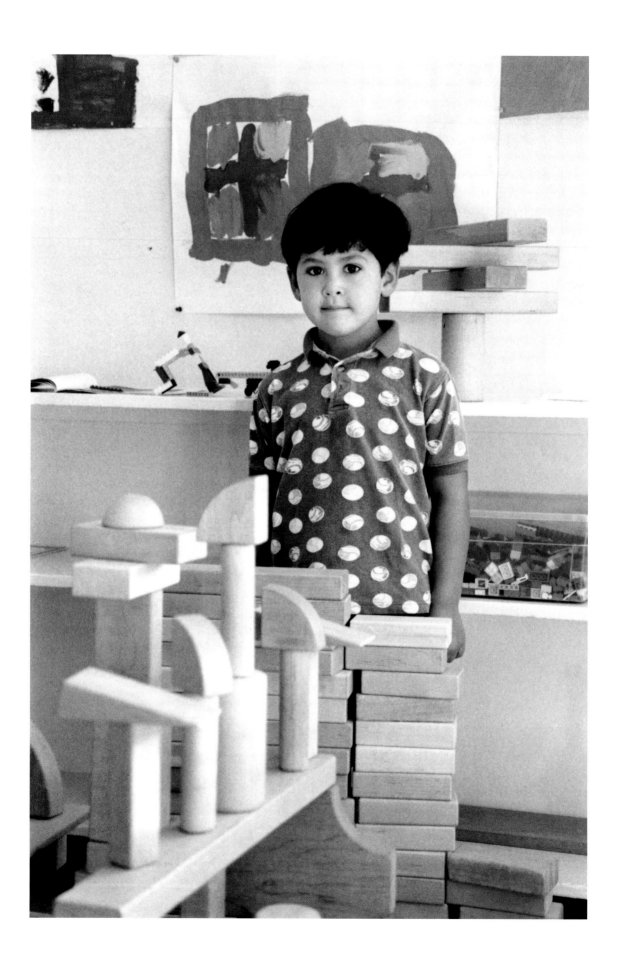

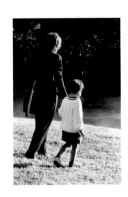

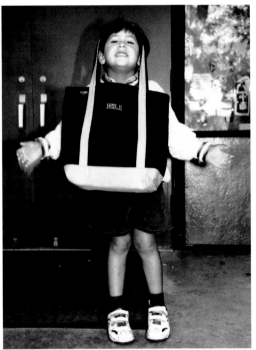

I'd like to get to that point
where they say the word "cure."
MARLENE

by eli
wn i gro up im goeng to be a arketat.
ef i kant be a arketat
il be a artst
ef i kant be a artst
il tri to be en the nba
bcas i lic to play baskitbil

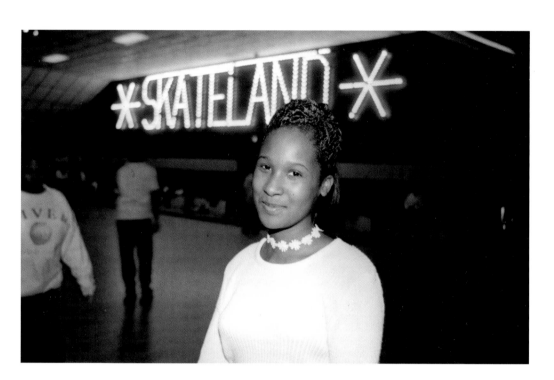

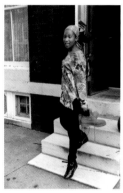

My hopes for Heather?

I want her to go to high school and be an athlete.

I want her to go to Spelman College.

I want her to be able to handle what's out there.

PHYLLIS

By the way, I want to be a model when I grow up.

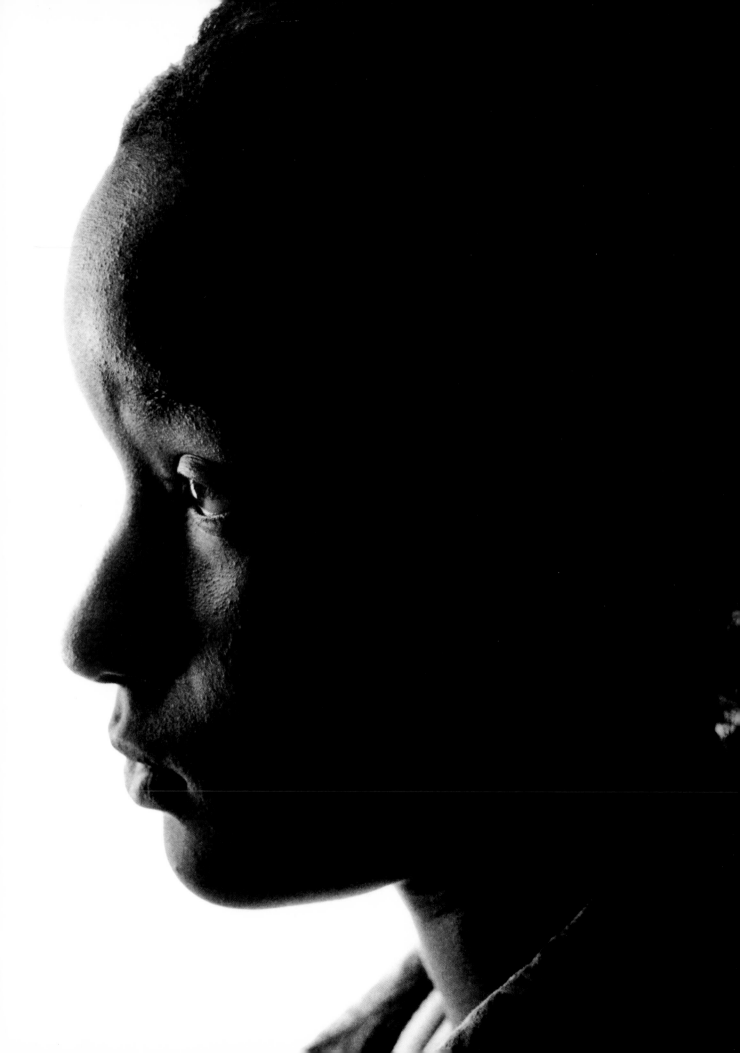

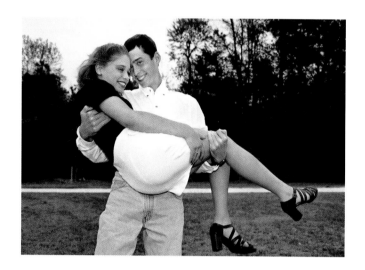

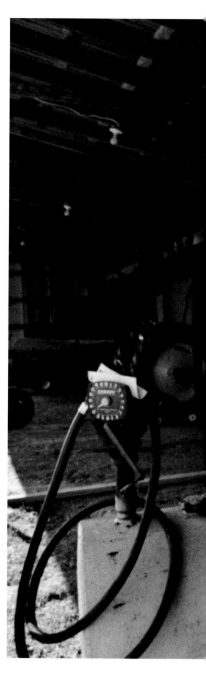

What good has come of this?

That he's alive.

Without the chemo, I would never have seen him dress up for the prom,

I would have never seen him be the best man at his brother's wedding,

I would not have seen him dressed up today for his new job.

> *The longer he lives the more memories I have—*
>
> *seeing him jumping on the trampoline or playing basketball.*
>
> *Look what he's been able to experience: he's got a beautiful girlfriend, great friends.*

> > *He's got so much now he didn't have then.*

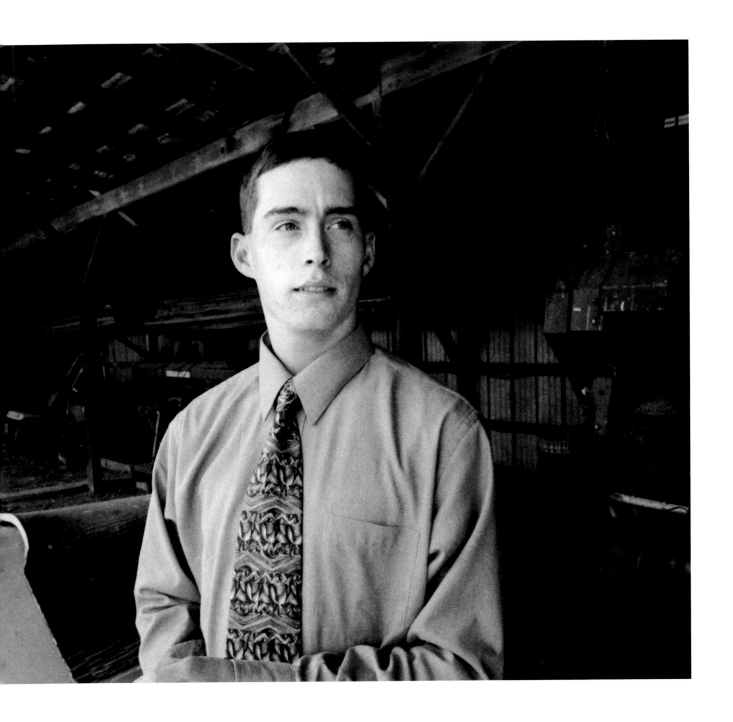

He's added on to his life. That is what living is about. You keep adding life. Every day.